THE CLEAN ABS FASCIA BOOK

Birds of a Feather

Chase Duquesnay EnQi Real

Amazon

This is dedicated to the dedicated.

CONTENTS

PREFACE

Thermogenic means tending to produce heat, and the term is commonly applied to drugs which increase heat through metabolic stimulation,[1] or to microorganisms which create heat within organic waste. Approximately all enzymatic reaction in the human body is thermogenic, which gives rise to the basal metabolic rate.[2]

In bodybuilding, athletes wishing to reduce body fat percentage use thermogenics in order to attempt to increase their basal metabolic rate, thereby increasing overall energy expenditure. Caffeine and ephedrine are commonly used for this purpose in the ECA stack. 2,4-Dinitrophenol (DNP) is a very strong thermogenic drug used for fat loss which produces a dose-dependent increase in body temperature, to the point where it can induce death by hyperthermia. It works as a mitochondrial oxidative phosphorylation uncoupler, disrupting the mitochondrial electron transport chain. This stops the mitochondria from producing adenosine triphosphate, causing energy to be released as heat.

There is a basic cost of energy to metabolize food. Carbohydrates are the cheapest, the fat and lastly protein.
Carbs cost about 5-15 percent of the energy the food gives you.

Fats cost about 10-20 percent of the energy the food gives you.

Proteins cost about 20-40 percent of the energy the food gives you.

Fiber rich veggies may be able to compete with Proteins, simply because they are water rich and give very few calories... they do take a good bit of energy to try and metabolize though...

This is important for Fat Burners, trying to build meal plans!

Think like this you look in your Divine Mathematics and Algarhythm books and see youve been doing 1000 calories of protein but your still losing weight...

Then you snap your finger and say "oh snap" I forgot that 20-40 percent of those calories vanish after eating. You thought you had 1000 calories of proteins, it was only 600-800... Get it?

Wait do not forget the Lemon I have lost whole humans worth of pounds with Lemons LOL....

Ok lets look at the body... and yes we have feathers, its official!

INTRODUCTION

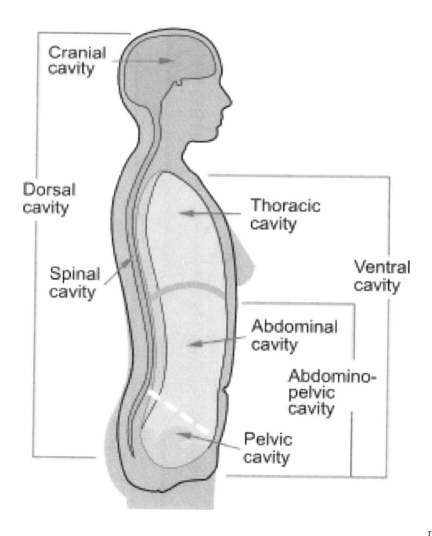

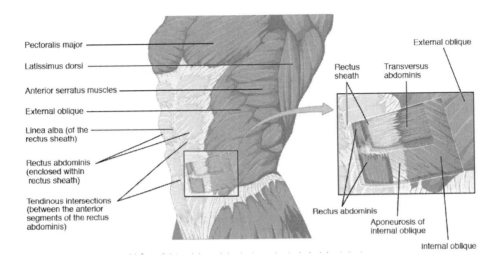

Pectoralis major

Latissimus dorsi

Anterior serratus muscles

External oblique

Linea alba (of the rectus sheath)

Rectus abdominis (enclosed within rectus sheath)

Tendinous intersections (between the anterior segments of the rectus abdominis)

External oblique

Rectus sheath

Transversus abdominis

Rectus abdominis

Aponeurosis of internal oblique

Internal oblique

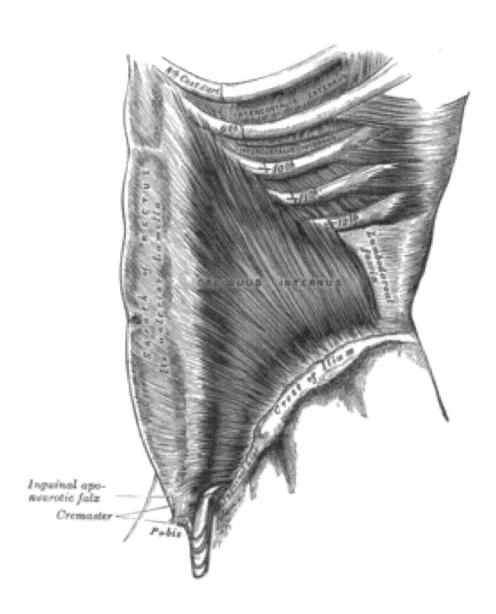

Inguinal apo-
neurotic falx

Cremaster

Pubis

Muscles of the Trunk

Pectoralis major

External oblique

Internal oblique

Rectus abdominis

Transverse abdominis

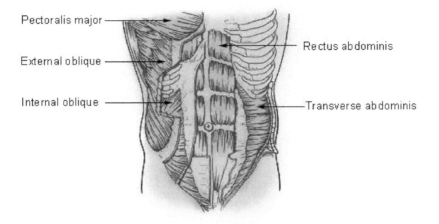

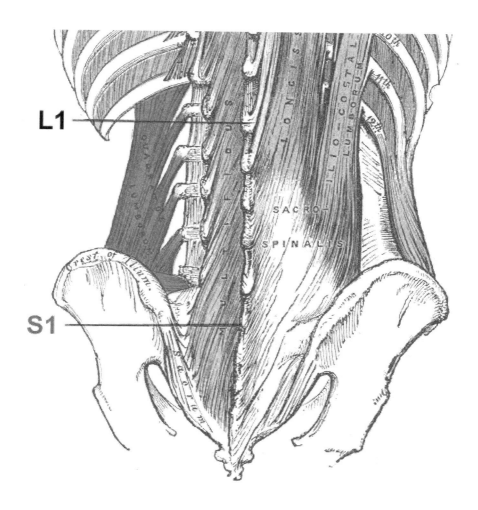

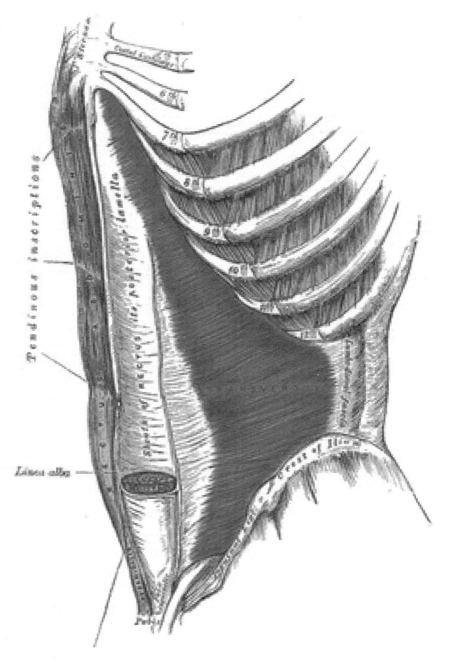

Tendinous Inscriptions

Linea alba

XIV

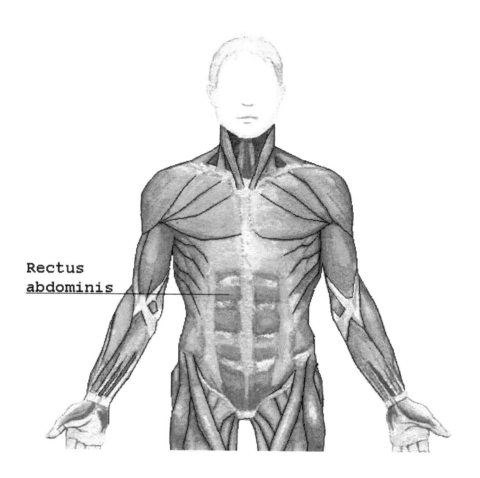

Rectus
abdominis

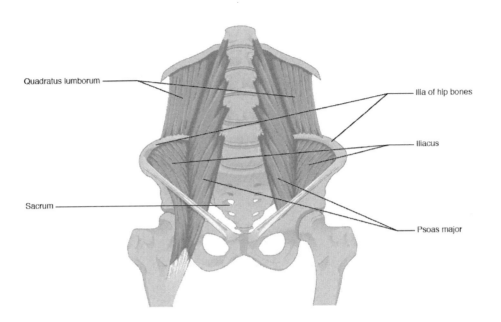

Quadratus lumborum

Ilia of hip bones

Iliacus

Sacrum

Psoas major

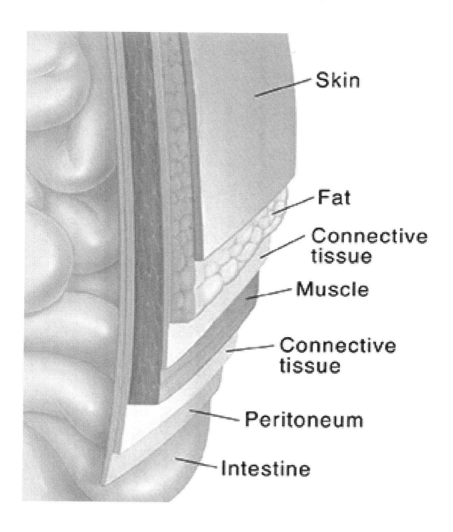

Skin

Fat

Connective tissue

Muscle

Connective tissue

Peritoneum

Intestine

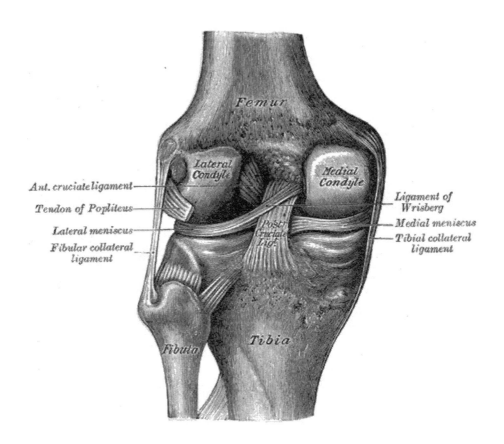

Femur

Lateral Condyle

Medial Condyle

Ant. cruciate ligament

Ligament of Wrisberg

Tendon of Popliteus

Medial meniscus

Lateral meniscus

Post. Cruciat. lig.

Tibial collateral ligament

Fibular collateral ligament

Fibula

Tibia

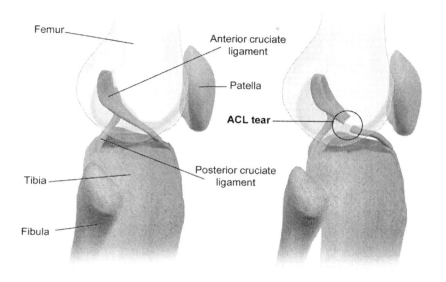

Femur

Anterior cruciate
ligament

Patella

ACL tear

Posterior cruciate
ligament

Tibia

Fibula

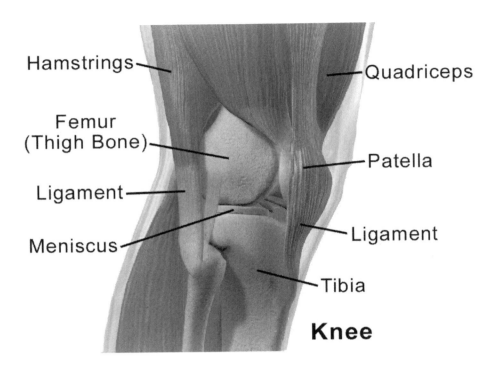

Hamstrings

Quadriceps

Femur
(Thigh Bone)

Patella

Ligament

Meniscus

Ligament

Tibia

Knee

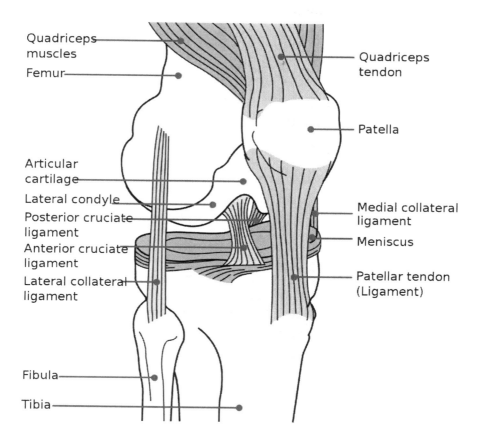

Quadriceps muscles

Femur

Articular cartilage

Lateral condyle

Posterior cruciate ligament

Anterior cruciate ligament

Lateral collateral ligament

Fibula

Tibia

Quadriceps tendon

Patella

Medial collateral ligament

Meniscus

Patellar tendon (Ligament)

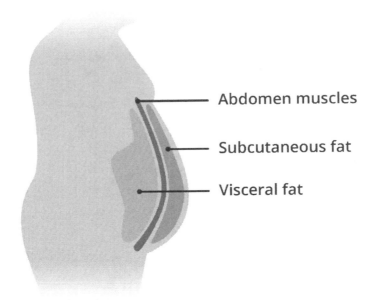

Abdomen muscles

Subcutaneous fat

Visceral fat

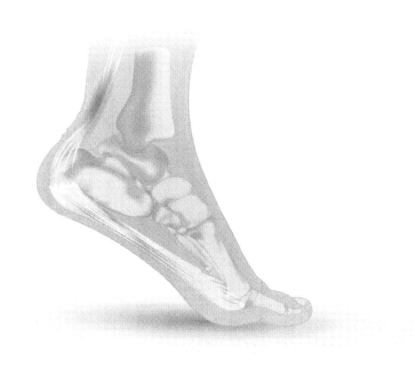

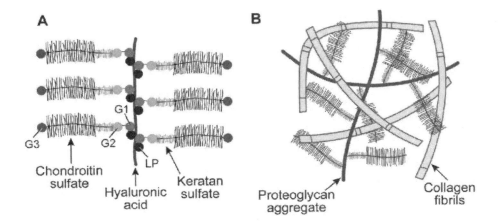

A

G1
G3
G2
LP
Chondroitin
sulfate
Hyaluronic
acid
Keratan
sulfate

B

Proteoglycan
aggregate
Collagen
fibrils

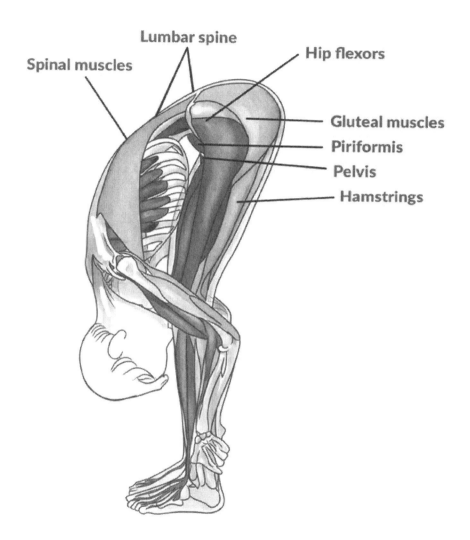

Lumbar spine

Spinal muscles

Hip flexors

Gluteal muscles

Piriformis

Pelvis

Hamstrings

Collagen fiber

Proteoglycan

CFPG complex

Collagenous tissue

Collagen
fibril

CFPG complex

GAG
duplex

Collagen
fiber

Interfibrillar failure

Protein
core

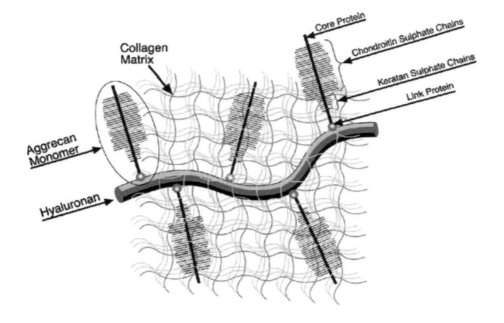

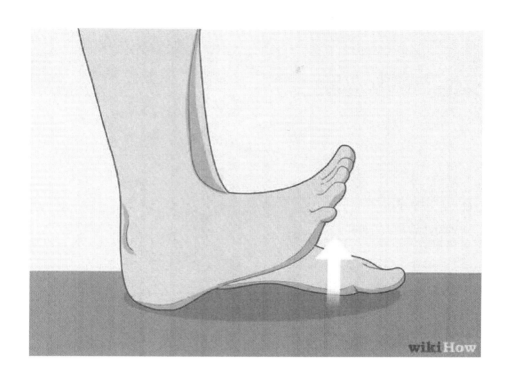

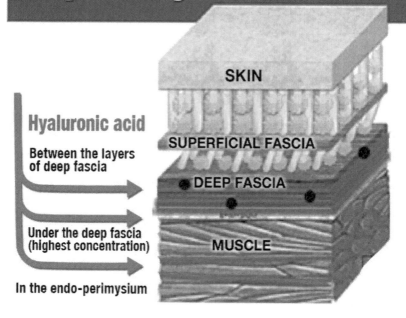

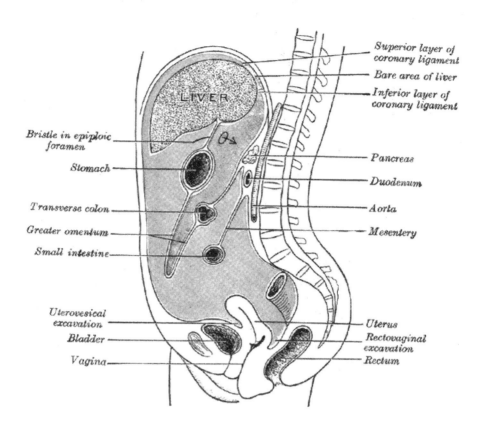

Superior layer of
coronary ligament

Bare area of liver

Inferior layer of
coronary ligament

LIVER

Bristle in epiploic
foramen

Stomach

Transverse colon

Greater omentum

Small intestine

Pancreas

Duodenum

Aorta

Mesentery

Uterovesical
excavation

Bladder

Vagina

Uterus

Rectovaginal
excavation

Rectum

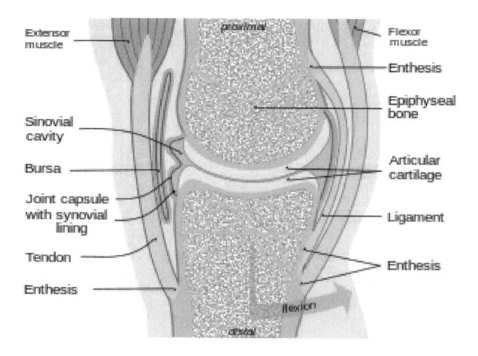

Extensor muscle

Flexor muscle

Enthesis

Epiphyseal bone

Sinovial cavity

Bursa

Articular cartilage

Joint capsule with synovial lining

Ligament

Tendon

Enthesis

Enthesis

proximal

flexion

distal

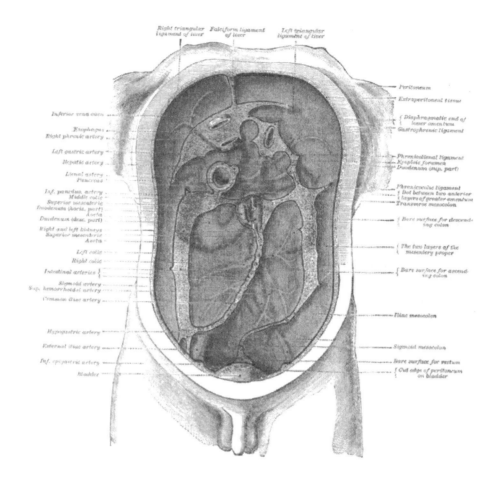

Right triangular ligament of liver   Falciform ligament of liver   Left triangular ligament of liver

Peritoneum

Extraperitoneal tissue

Inferior vena cava

Diaphragmatic end of lesser omentum
Gastrophrenic ligament

Œsophagus
Right phrenic artery

Left gastric artery

Phrenicolienal ligament
Epiploic foramen
Duodenum (sup. part)

Hepatic artery

Lienal artery
Pancreas

Phrenicocolic ligament
Bet between two anterior layers of greater omentum
Transverse mesocolon

Inf. pancreatic artery
Middle colic
Superior mesenteric
Duodenum (horiz. part)
Aorta
Duodenum (desc. part)

Bare surface for descending colon

Right and left kidneys
Superior mesenteric
Aorta

The two layers of the mesentery proper

Left colic

Right colic

Intestinal arteries {

Bare surface for ascending colon

Sigmoid artery
Sup. hæmorrhoidal artery

Common iliac artery

Iliac mesocolon

Hypogastric artery

Sigmoid mesocolon

External iliac artery

Bare surface for rectum

Inf. epigastric artery

Cut edge of peritoneum on bladder

Bladder

XXXIII

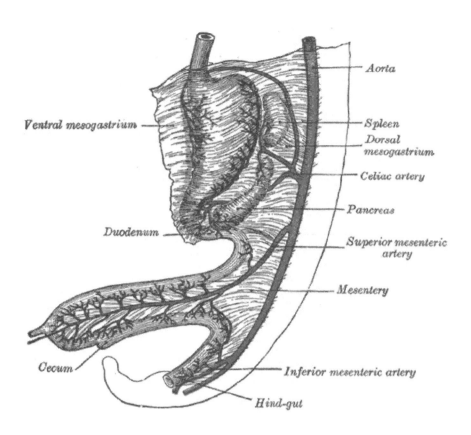

Ventral mesogastrium

Duodenum

Cecum

Aorta

Spleen

Dorsal
mesogastrium

Celiac artery

Pancreas

Superior mesenteric
artery

Mesentery

Inferior mesenteric artery

Hind-gut

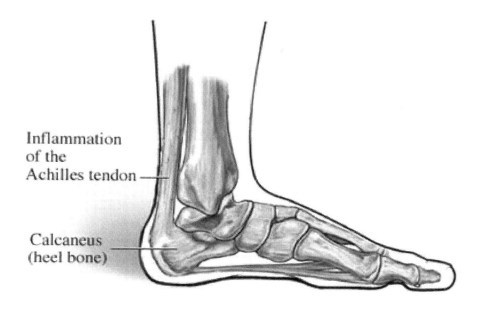

Inflammation
of the
Achilles tendon

Calcaneus
(heel bone)

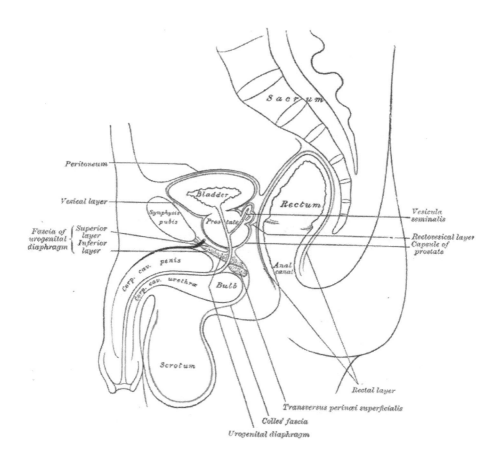

Peritoneum

Vesical layer

Fascia of
urogenital
diaphragm { Superior
layer
Inferior
layer

Sacrum

Bladder

Symphysis
pubis

Prostate

Rectum

Corp. cav. penis

Corp. cav. urethra

Bulb

Anal
canal

Vesicula
seminalis

Rectovesical layer
Capsule of
prostate

Scrotum

Rectal layer

Transversus perinæi superficialis

Colles' fascia

Urogenital diaphragm

XXXVI

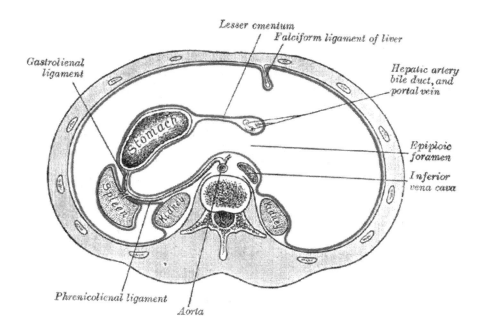

Lesser omentum

Falciform ligament of liver

Gastrolienal ligament

Hepatic artery bile duct, and portal vein

Stomach

Epiploic foramen

Inferior vena cava

Spleen

Kidney

Kidney

Phrenicolienal ligament

Aorta

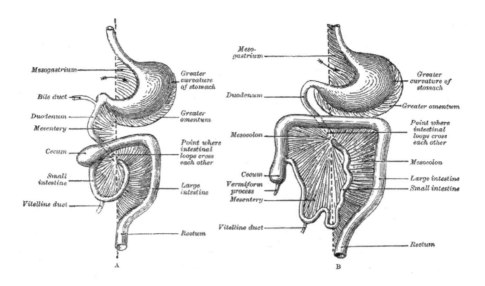

Mesogastrium

Bile duct

Duodenum

Mesentery

Cecum

Small
intestine

Vitelline duct

Greater
curvature
of stomach

Greater
omentum

Point where
intestinal
loops cross
each other

Large
intestine

Rectum

A

Meso-
gastrium

Duodenum

Mesocolon

Cecum

Vermiform
process

Mesentery

Vitelline duct

Greater
curvature of
stomach

Greater omentum

Point where
intestinal
loops cross
each other

Mesocolon

Large intestine

Small intestine

Rectum

B

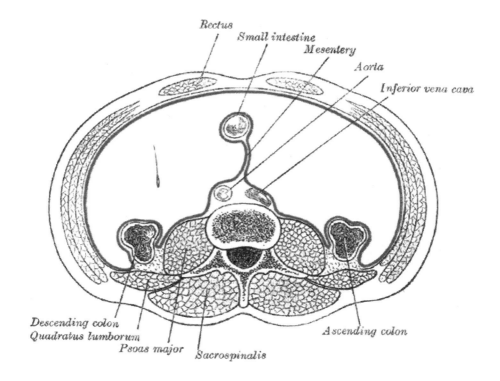

Rectus

Small intestine

Mesentery

Aorta

Inferior vena cava

Descending colon
Quadratus lumborum
Psoas major
Sacrospinalis
Ascending colon

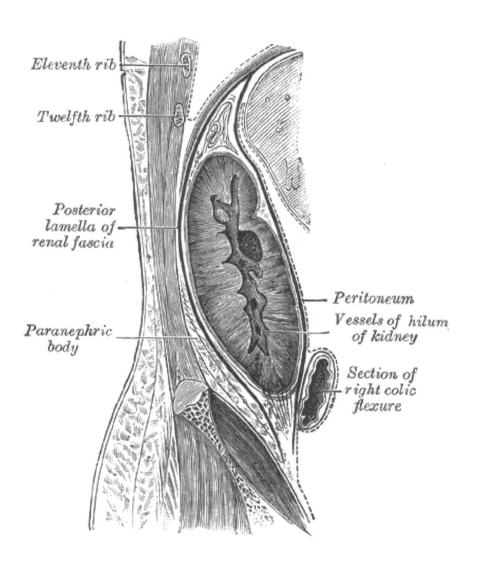

Eleventh rib

Twelfth rib

Posterior lamella of renal fascia

Paranephric body

Peritoneum

Vessels of hilum of kidney

Section of right colic flexure

XL

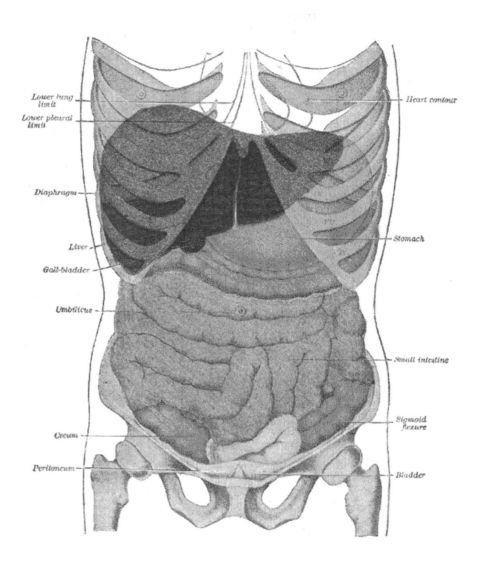

Lower lung
limit

Lower pleural
limit

Diaphragm

Liver

Gall-bladder

Umbilicus

Cæcum

Peritoneum

Heart contour

Stomach

Small intestine

Sigmoid
flexure

Bladder

XLI

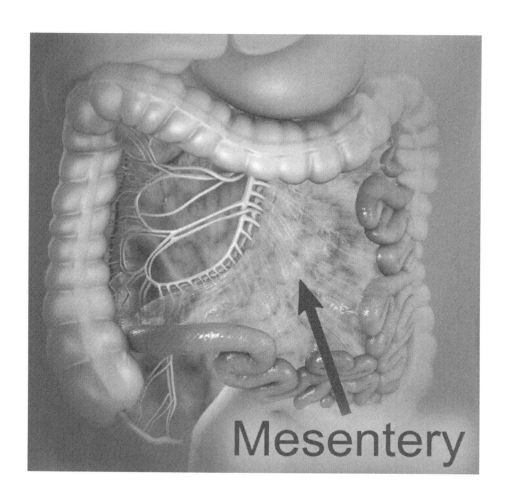

Mesentery

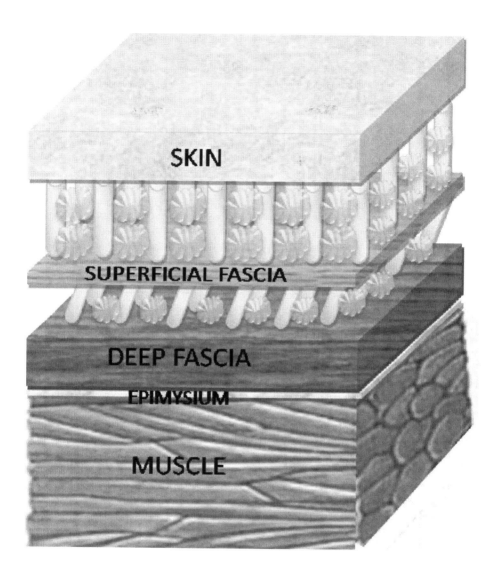

SKIN

SUPERFICIAL FASCIA

DEEP FASCIA

EPIMYSIUM

MUSCLE

FISH SCALE

Did you know that as embryos we have gills? Why? Not why did you know or not, but why do we have them? Were our ancestors telling us needed science in the Animal God stories or were they just doing Cosplay?

The **Cambrian explosion** (also known as **Cambrian radiation**[1] or **Cambrian diversification**) is an interval of time approximately 538.8 million years ago in the Cambrian period of the early Paleozoic when there was a sudden radiation of complex life, and practically all major animal phyla started appearing in the fossil record.[2][3][4] It lasted for about 13[5][6][7] to 25[8][9] million years and resulted in the divergence of most modern metazoan phyla.[10] The event was accompanied by major diversification in other groups of organisms as well.[a]

Before early Cambrian diversification,[b] most organisms were relatively simple, composed of individual cells, or small multicellular organisms, occasionally organized into colonies. As the rate of diversification subsequently accelerated, the variety of life became much more complex, and began to resemble that of today.[12] Almost all present-day animal phyla appeared during this period,[13][14] including the earliest chordates.[15]

A 2019 paper suggests that the timing should be expanded back to include the late Ediacaran, where another diverse soft-bodied biota existed and possibly persisted into the Cambrian, rather than just the narrower timeframe of the "Cambrian Explosion" event visible in the fossil record, based on analysis of chemicals that would have laid the building blocks for a progression of transitional radiations starting with the Ediacaran period and continuing at a similar rate into the Cambrian.[16]

Key Cambrian explosion events

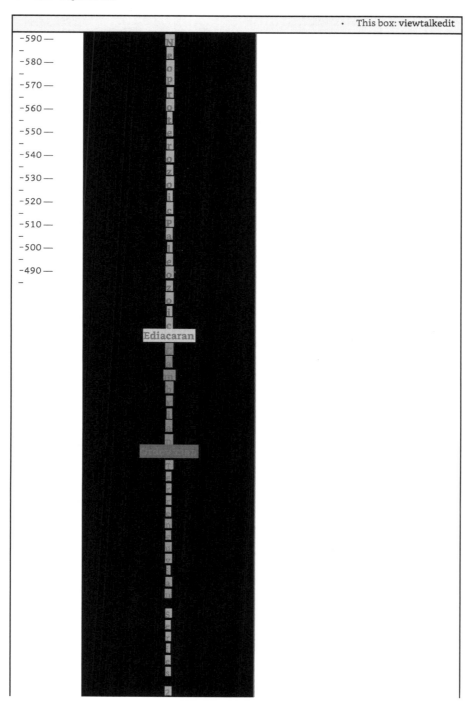

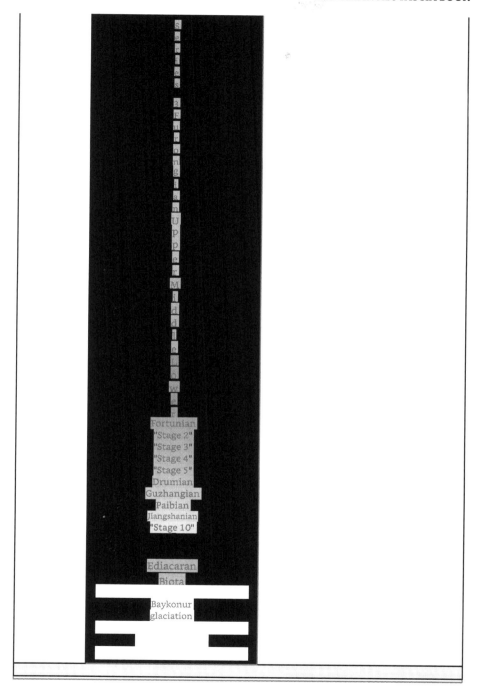

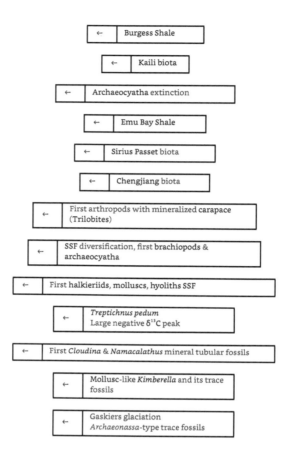

History and significance[edit]

Life timeline
· This box: viewtalkedit

−4500 —	Water
−	
—	Single-celled life
−	
−4000 —	Photosynthesis
−	
—	
—	Eukaryotes
−	
−3500 —	Multicellular life
−	
—	
−	P
−3000 —	l
−	

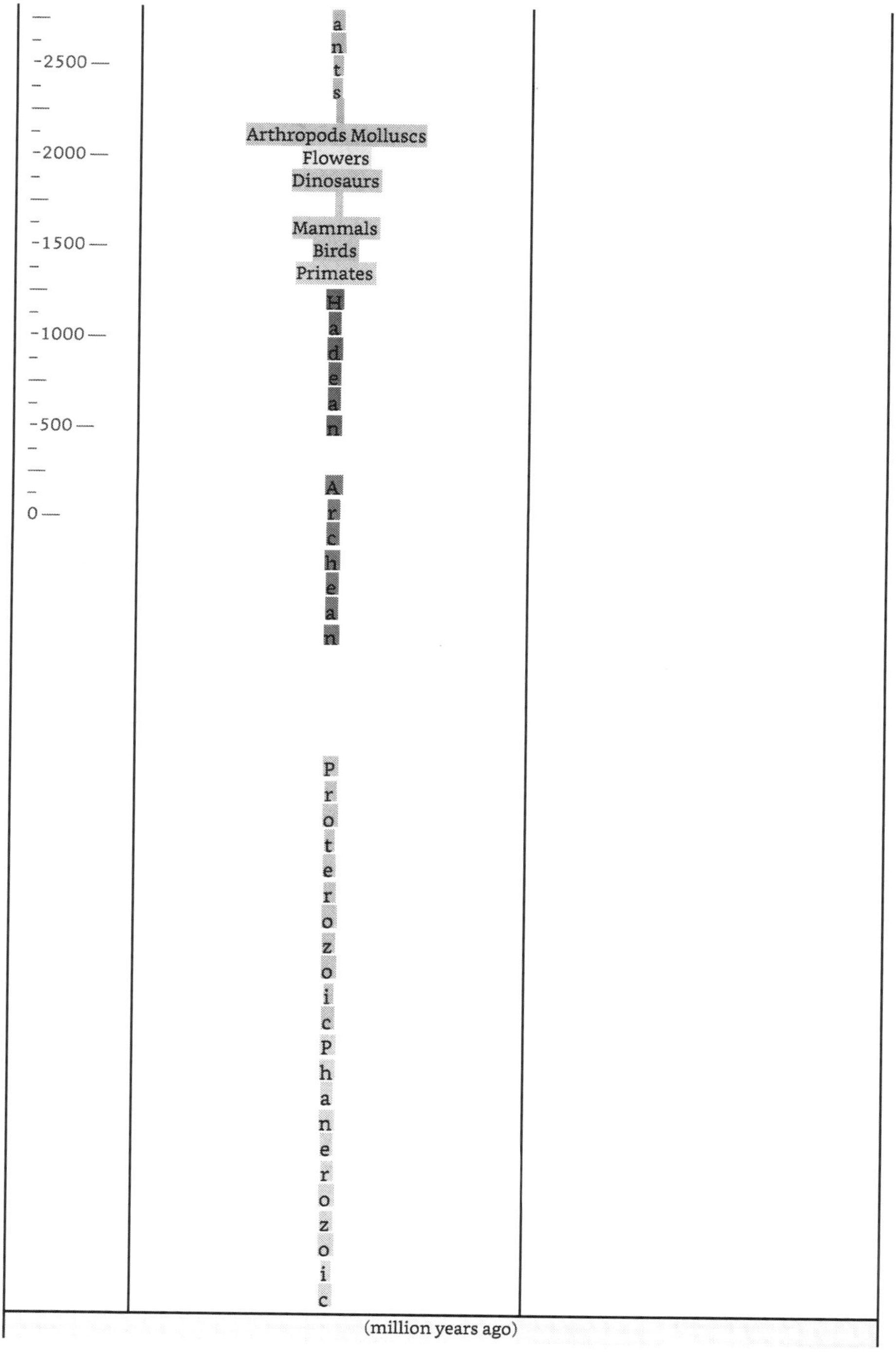

-2500 —

-2000 —

-1500 —

-1000 —

-500 —

0 —

ants

Arthropods Molluscs
Flowers
Dinosaurs

Mammals
Birds
Primates

Hadean

Archean

Proterozoic Phanerozoic

(million years ago)

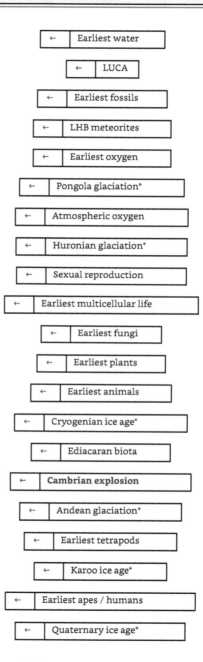

*Ice Ages

Earliest water

LUCA

Earliest fossils

LHB meteorites

Earliest oxygen

Pongola glaciation*

Atmospheric oxygen

Huronian glaciation*

Sexual reproduction

Earliest multicellular life

Earliest fungi

Earliest plants

Earliest animals

Cryogenian ice age*

Ediacaran biota

Cambrian explosion

Andean glaciation*

Earliest tetrapods

Karoo ice age*

Earliest apes / humans

Quaternary ice age*

Main article: History of life

The seemingly rapid appearance of fossils in the "Primordial Strata" was noted by William Buckland in the 1840s,[17] and in his 1859 book On the Origin of Species, Charles Darwin discussed the then-inexplicable lack of earlier fossils as one of the main difficulties for his theory of descent with slow modification through natural selection.[18] The long-running puzzlement about the seemingly-sudden appearance of the Cambrian fauna without evident precursor(s) centers on three key points: whether there really was a mass diversification of complex organisms over a relatively short period during the early Cambrian, what might have caused such rapid change, and what it would imply about the origin of animal life. Interpretation is difficult, owing to a limited supply of evidence based mainly on an incomplete fossil record and chemical signatures remaining in Cambrian rocks.

The first discovered Cambrian fossils were trilobites, described by Edward Lhuyd, the curator of Oxford Museum, in 1698. [19] Although their evolutionary importance was not known, on the basis of their old age, William Buckland (1784–1856) realized that a dramatic step-change in the fossil record had occurred around the base of what we now call the Cambrian.[17] Nineteenth-century geologists such as Adam Sedgwick and Roderick Murchison used the fossils for dating rock strata, specifically for establishing the Cambrian and Silurian periods.[20] By 1859, leading geologists including Roderick Murchison were convinced that what was then called the lowest Silurian stratum showed the origin of life on Earth, though others, including Charles Lyell, differed. In On the Origin of Species, Darwin considered this sudden appearance of a solitary group of trilobites, with no apparent antecedents, and absent other fossils, to be "undoubtedly of the gravest nature" among the difficulties in his theory of natural selection. He reasoned that earlier seas had swarmed with living creatures, but that their fossils had not been found because of the imperfections of the fossil record.[18] In the sixth edition of his book, he stressed his problem further as:[21]

To the question why we do not find rich fossiliferous deposits belonging to these assumed earliest periods prior to the Cambrian system, I can give no satisfactory answer.

American paleontologist Charles Walcott, who studied the Burgess Shale fauna, proposed that an interval of time, the "Lipalian", was not represented in the fossil record or did not preserve fossils, and that the ancestors of the Cambrian animals evolved during this time.[22]

Earlier fossil evidence has since been found. The earliest claim is that the history of life on Earth goes back 3,850 million years:[23] Rocks of that age at Warrawoona, Australia, were claimed to contain fossil stromatolites, stubby pillars formed by colonies of microorganisms. Fossils (Grypania) of more complex eukaryotic cells, from which all animals, plants, and fungi are built, have been found in rocks from 1,400 million years ago, in China and Montana. Rocks dating from 580 to 543 million years ago contain fossils of the Ediacara biota, organisms so large that they are likely multicelled, but very unlike any modern organism. [24] In 1948, Preston Cloud argued that a period of "eruptive" evolution occurred in the Early Cambrian,[25] but as recently as the 1970s, no sign was seen of how the 'relatively' modern-looking organisms of the Middle and Late Cambrian arose.[24]

Opabinia made the largest single contribution to modern interest in the Cambrian explosion.

The intense modern interest in this "Cambrian explosion" was sparked by the work of Harry B. Whittington and colleagues, who, in the 1970s, reanalysed many fossils from the Burgess Shale and concluded that several were as complex as, but different from, any living animals.[26][27] The most common organism, Marrella, was clearly an arthropod, but not a member of any known arthropod class. Organisms such as the five-eyed Opabinia and spiny slug-like Wiwaxia were so different from anything else known that Whittington's team assumed they must represent different phyla, seemingly unrelated to anything known today. Stephen Jay Gould's popular 1989 account of this work, Wonderful Life,[28] brought the matter into the public eye and raised questions about what the explosion represented. While differing significantly in details, both Whittington and Gould proposed that all modern animal phyla had appeared almost simultaneously in a rather short span of geological period. This view led to the modernization of Darwin's tree of life and the theory of punctuated equilibrium, which Eldredge and Gould developed in the early 1970s and which views evolution as long intervals of near-stasis "punctuated" by short periods of rapid change.[29]

Other analyses, some more recent and some dating back to the 1970s, argue that complex animals similar to modern types evolved well before the start of the Cambrian.[30][31][32]

Dating the Cambrian[edit]

Radiometric dates for much of the Cambrian, obtained by analysis of radioactive elements contained within rocks, have only recently become available, and for only a few regions.

Relative dating (A was before B) is often assumed sufficient for studying processes of evolution, but this, too, has been difficult, because of the problems involved in matching up rocks of the same age across different continents.[33]

Therefore, dates or descriptions of sequences of events should be regarded with some caution until better data become available. In 2004, the start of the Cambrian was dated to 542 Ma.[34] In 2012, it was revised to 541 Ma[35] then in 2022 it was changed again to 538.8 Ma.[2] Some theory suggest Cambrian explosion occurred during the last stages of Gondwanan assembly, which is formed following Rodinia splitting, overlapped with the opening of the Iapetus Ocean between Laurentia and western Gondwana.[36][37] The largest Cambrian faunal province is located around Gondwana, which extended from the low northern latitudes to the high southern latitudes, just short of the South Pole. By the middle and later parts of the Cambrian, continued rifting had sent the paleocontinents of Laurentia, Baltica and Siberia on their separate ways.[38]

Body fossils[edit]

Fossils of organisms' bodies are usually the most informative type of evidence. Fossilization is a rare event, and most fossils are destroyed by erosion or metamorphism before they can be observed. Hence, the fossil record is very incomplete, increasingly so as earlier times are considered. Despite this, they are often adequate to illustrate the broader patterns of life's history.[39] Also, biases exist in the fossil record: different environments are more favourable to the preservation of different types of organism or parts of organisms.[40] Further, only the parts of organisms that were already mineralised are usually preserved, such as the shells of molluscs. Since most animal species are soft-bodied, they decay before they can become fossilised. As a result, although 30-plus phyla of living animals are known, two-thirds have never been found as fossils.[24]

This Marrella specimen illustrates how clear and detailed the fossils from the Burgess Shale Lagerstätte actually are as well as the oldest evidence for liquid blood in an animal.

The Cambrian fossil record includes an unusually high number of lagerstätten, which preserve soft tissues. These allow paleontologists to examine the internal anatomy of animals, which in other sediments are only represented by shells, spines, claws, etc. – if they are preserved at all. The most significant Cambrian lagerstätten are the early Cambrian Maotianshan shale beds of Chengjiang (Yunnan, China) and Sirius Passet (Greenland);[41] the middle Cambrian Burgess Shale (British Columbia, Canada);[42] and the late Cambrian Orsten (Sweden) fossil beds.

While lagerstätten preserve far more than the conventional fossil record, they are far from complete. Because lagerstätten are restricted to a narrow range of environments (where soft-bodied organisms can be preserved very quickly, e.g. by mudslides), most animals are probably not represented; further, the exceptional conditions that create lagerstätten probably do not represent normal living conditions. [43] In addition, the known Cambrian lagerstätten are rare and difficult to date, while Precambrian lagerstätten have yet to be studied in detail. The sparseness of the fossil record means that organisms usually exist long before they are found in the fossil record – this is known as the Signor–Lipps effect.[44]

In 2019, a "stunning" find of lagerstätten, known as the Qingjiang biota, was reported from the Danshui river in Hubei province, China. More than 20,000 fossil specimens were collected, including many soft bodied animals such as jellyfish, sea anemones and worms, as well as sponges, arthropods and algae. In some specimens the internal body structures were sufficiently preserved that soft tissues, including muscles, gills, mouths, guts and eyes, can be seen. The remains were dated to around 518 Mya and around half of the species identified at the time of reporting were previously unknown.[45][46][47]

Trace fossils[edit]

Rusophycus and other trace fossils from the Gog Group, Middle Cambrian, Lake Louise, Alberta, Canada

Trace fossils consist mainly of tracks and burrows, but also include coprolites (fossil feces) and marks left by feeding.[48][49] Trace fossils are particularly significant because they represent a data source that is not limited to animals with easily fossilized hard parts, and reflects organisms' behaviour. Also, many traces date from significantly earlier than the body fossils of animals that are thought to have been capable of making them.[50] While exact assignment of trace fossils to their makers is generally impossible, traces may, for example, provide the earliest physical evidence of the appearance of moderately complex animals (comparable to earthworms).[49]

Geochemical observations[edit]

Main article: Early Cambrian geochemical fluctuations

Several chemical markers indicate a drastic change in the environment around the start of the Cambrian. The markers are consistent with a mass extinction,[51][52] or with a massive warming resulting from the release of methane ice.[53] Such changes may reflect a cause of the Cambrian explosion, although they may also have resulted from an increased level of biological activity – a possible result of the explosion. [53] Despite these uncertainties, the geochemical evidence helps by making scientists focus on theories that are consistent with at least one of the likely environmental changes.

Phylogenetic techniques[edit]

Cladistics is a technique for working out the "family tree" of a set of organisms. It works by the logic that, if groups B and C have more similarities to each other than either has to group A, then B and C are more closely related to each other than either is to A. Characteristics that are compared may be anatomical, such as the presence of a notochord, or molecular, by comparing sequences of DNA or protein. The result of a successful analysis is a hierarchy of clades – groups whose members are believed to share a common ancestor. The cladistic technique is sometimes problematic, as some features, such as wings or camera eyes, evolved more than once, convergently – this must be taken into account in analyses.

From the relationships, it may be possible to constrain the date that lineages first appeared. For instance, if fossils of B or C date to X million years ago and the calculated "family tree" says A was an ancestor of B and C, then A must have evolved more than X million years ago.

It is also possible to estimate how long ago two living clades diverged – i.e. about how long ago their last common ancestor must have lived – by assuming that DNA mutations accumulate at a constant rate. These "molecular clocks", however, are fallible, and provide only a very approximate timing: they are not sufficiently precise and reliable for estimating when the groups that feature in the Cambrian explosion first evolved,[54] and estimates produced by different techniques vary by a factor of two.[55] However, the clocks can give an indication of branching rate, and when combined with the constraints of the fossil record, recent clocks suggest a sustained period of diversification through the Ediacaran and Cambrian.[56]

Explanation of key scientific terms[edit]

Stem groups[57]

- — = Lines of descent
- = Basal node
- = Crown node

- = Total group
- = Crown group
- = Stem group

Phylum[edit]

A phylum is the highest level in the Linnaean system for classifying organisms. Phyla can be thought of as groupings of animals based on general body plan.[58] Despite the seemingly different external appearances of organisms, they are classified into phyla based on their internal and developmental organizations.[59] For example, despite their obvious differences, spiders and barnacles both belong to the phylum Arthropoda, but earthworms and tapeworms, although similar in shape, belong to different phyla. As chemical and genetic testing becomes more accurate, previously hypothesised phyla are often entirely reworked.

A phylum is not a fundamental division of nature, such as the difference between electrons and protons. It is simply a very high-level grouping in a classification system created to describe all currently living organisms. This system is imperfect, even for modern animals: different books quote different numbers of phyla, mainly because they disagree about the classification of a huge number of worm-like species. As it is based on living organisms, it accommodates extinct organisms poorly, if at all.[24][60]

Stem group[edit]

The concept of stem groups was introduced to cover evolutionary "aunts" and "cousins" of living groups, and have been hypothesized based on this scientific theory. A crown group is a group of closely related living animals plus their last common ancestor plus all its descendants. A stem group is a set of offshoots from the lineage at a point earlier than the last common ancestor of the crown group; it is a relative concept, for example tardigrades are living animals that form a crown group in their own right, but Budd (1996) regarded them as also being a stem group relative to the arthropods.[57][61]

Skin
(ectoderm)
Muscle
(mesoderm)
Coelom
Internal

organ

Membrane
(peritoneum)

Gut
(endoderm)

A coelomate animal is basically a set of concentric tubes, with a gap between the gut and the outer tubes.

Triploblastic[edit]

The term Triploblastic means consisting of three layers, which are formed in the embryo, quite early in the animal's development from a single-celled egg to a larva or juvenile form. The innermost layer forms the digestive tract (gut); the outermost forms skin; and the middle one forms muscles and all the internal organs except the digestive system. Most types of living animal are triploblastic – the best-known exceptions are Porifera (sponges) and Cnidaria (jellyfish, sea anemones, etc.).

Bilaterian[edit]

The bilaterians are animals that have right and left sides at some point in their life histories. This implies that they have top and bottom surfaces and, importantly, distinct front and back ends. All known bilaterian animals are triploblastic, and all known triploblastic animals are bilaterian. Living echinoderms (sea stars, sea urchins, sea cucumbers, etc.) 'look' radially symmetrical (like wheels) rather than bilaterian, but their larvae exhibit bilateral symmetry and some of the earliest echinoderms may have been bilaterally symmetrical.[62] Porifera and Cnidaria are radially symmetrical, not bilaterian, and not triploblastic (but the common Bilateria-Cnidaria ancestor's planula larva is suspected to be bilaterally symmetric).

Coelomate[edit]

The term Coelomate means having a body cavity (coelom) containing the internal organs. Most of the phyla featured in the debate about the Cambrian explosion[clarification needed] are coelomates: arthropods, annelid worms, molluscs, echinoderms, and chordates – the noncoelomate priapulids are an important exception. All known coelomate animals are triploblastic bilaterians, but some triploblastic bilaterian animals do not have a coelom – for example flatworms, whose organs are surrounded by unspecialized tissues.

Precambrian life[edit]

Evidence of animals around 1 billion years ago[edit]

Further information: Acritarch and Stromatolite

Stromatolites (Pika Formation, Middle Cambrian) near Helen Lake, Banff National Park, Canada

Modern stromatolites in Hamelin Pool Marine Nature Reserve, Western Australia

Changes in the abundance and diversity of some types of fossil have been interpreted as evidence for "attacks" by animals or other organisms. Stromatolites, stubby pillars built by colonies of microorganisms, are a major constituent of the fossil record from about 2,700 million years ago, but their abundance and diversity declined steeply after about 1,250 million years ago. This decline has been attributed to disruption by grazing and burrowing animals.[30][31][63]

Precambrian marine diversity was dominated by small fossils known as acritarchs. This term describes almost any small organic walled fossil – from the egg cases of small metazoans to resting cysts of many different kinds of green algae. After appearing around 2,000 million years ago, acritarchs underwent a boom around 1,000 million years ago, increasing in abundance, diversity, size, complexity of shape, and especially size and number of spines. Their increasingly spiny forms in the last 1 billion years may indicate an increased need for defence against predation. Other groups of small organisms from the Neoproterozoic era also show signs of antipredator defenses.[63] A consideration of taxon longevity appears to support an increase in predation pressure around this time.[64]

In general, the fossil record shows a very slow appearance of these lifeforms in the Precambrian, with many cyanobacterial species making up much of the underlying sediment.

An Ediacaran trace fossil, made when an organism burrowed below a microbial mat.

Ediacaran organisms[edit]

Dickinsonia costata, an Ediacaran organism of unknown affinity, with a quilted appearance

Main articles: Ediacaran biota, Cloudinidae, Kimberella, and Spriggina

At the start of the Ediacaran period, much of the acritarch fauna, which had remained relatively unchanged for hundreds of millions of years, became extinct, to be replaced with a range of new, larger species, which would prove far more ephemeral.[65] This radiation, the first in the fossil record,[65] is followed soon after by an array of unfamiliar, large

14

fossils dubbed the Ediacara biota,[66] which flourished for 40 million years until the start of the Cambrian.[67] Most of this "Ediacara biota" were at least a few centimeters long, significantly larger than any earlier fossils. The organisms form three distinct assemblages, increasing in size and complexity as time progressed.[68]

Many of these organisms were quite unlike anything that appeared before or since, resembling discs, mud-filled bags, or quilted mattresses – one paleontologist proposed that the strangest organisms should be classified as a separate kingdom, Vendozoa.[69]

Fossil of Kimberella, a triploblastic bilaterian, and possibly a mollusc

At least some may have been early forms of the phyla at the heart of the "Cambrian explosion" debate,[clarification needed] having been interpreted as early molluscs (Kimberella), [32][70] echinoderms (Arkarua);[71] and arthropods (Spriggina, [72] Parvancorina,[73] Yilingia). Still, debate exists about the classification of these specimens, mainly because the diagnostic features that allow taxonomists to classify more recent organisms, such as similarities to living organisms, are generally absent in the ediacarans.[74] However, there seems little doubt that Kimberella was at least a triploblastic bilaterian animal.[74] These organisms are central to the debate about how abrupt the Cambrian explosion was. [citation needed] If some were early members of the animal phyla seen today, the "explosion" looks a lot less sudden than if all these organisms represent an unrelated "experiment", and were replaced by the animal kingdom fairly soon thereafter (40M years is "soon" by evolutionary and geological standards).

The traces of organisms moving on and directly underneath the microbial mats that covered the Ediacaran sea floor are preserved from the Ediacaran period, about 565 million years ago.[c] They were probably made by organisms resembling earthworms in shape, size, and how they moved. The burrow-makers have never been found preserved, but, because they would need a head and a tail, the burrowers probably had bilateral symmetry – which would in all probability make them bilaterian animals.[77] They fed above the sediment surface, but were forced to burrow to avoid predators.[78]

Cambrian life[edit]

Trace fossils[edit]

Trace fossils (burrows, etc.) are a reliable indicator of what life was around, and indicate a diversification of life around the start of the Cambrian, with the freshwater realm colonized by animals almost as quickly as the oceans.[79]

Small shelly fauna[edit]

Main article: Small shelly fauna

Fossils known as "small shelly fauna" have been found in many parts on the world, and date from just before the Cambrian to about 10 million years after the start of the Cambrian (the Nemakit-Daldynian and Tommotian ages; see timeline). These are a very mixed collection of fossils: spines, sclerites (armor plates), tubes, archeocyathids (sponge-like animals), and small shells very like those of brachiopods and snail-like molluscs – but all tiny, mostly 1 to 2 mm long.[80]

While small, these fossils are far more common than complete fossils of the organisms that produced them; crucially, they cover the window from the start of the Cambrian to the first lagerstätten: a period of time otherwise lacking in fossils. Hence, they supplement the conventional fossil record and allow the fossil ranges of many groups to be extended.

Cnidarians[edit]

The first cnidarian larvae, represented by the genus Eolarva, appeared in the Cambrian, although the identity of Eolarva as such is controversial. If it does represent a cnidarian larva, Eolarva would represent the first fossil evidence of indirect development in metazoans in the earliest Cambrian.[81]

Medusozoans developed complex life cycles with a medusa stage during the Cambrian explosion, as evidenced by the discovery of Burgessomedusa phasmiformis.[82]

Trilobites[edit]

A fossilized trilobite, an ancient type of arthropod: This specimen, from the Burgess Shale, preserves "soft parts" – the antennae and legs.

The earliest trilobite fossils are about 530 million years old, but the class was already quite diverse and cosmopolitan, suggesting they had been around for quite some time.[83] The fossil record of trilobites began with the appearance of trilobites with mineral exoskeletons – not from the time of their origin.

Crustaceans[edit]

Further information: Orsten

Crustaceans, one of the four great modern groups of arthropods, are very rare throughout the Cambrian. Convincing crustaceans were once thought to be common in Burgess Shale-type biotas, but none of these individuals can be shown to fall into the crown group of "true crustaceans".[84] The Cambrian record of crown-group crustaceans comes from microfossils. The Swedish Orsten horizons contain later Cambrian crustaceans, but only organisms smaller than 2 mm are preserved. This restricts the data set to juveniles and miniaturised adults.

A more informative data source is the organic microfossils of the Mount Cap formation, Mackenzie Mountains, Canada. This late Early Cambrian assemblage (510 to 515 million years ago) consists of microscopic fragments of arthropods' cuticle, which is left behind when the rock is dissolved with hydrofluoric acid. The diversity of this assemblage is similar to that of modern crustacean faunas. Analysis of fragments of feeding machinery found in the formation shows that it was adapted to feed in a very precise and refined fashion. This contrasts with most other early Cambrian arthropods, which fed messily by shovelling anything they could get their feeding appendages on into their mouths. This sophisticated and specialised feeding machinery belonged to a large (about 30 cm)[85] organism, and would have provided great potential for diversification: Specialised feeding apparatus allows a number of different approaches to feeding and development, and creates a number of different approaches to avoid being eaten.[84]

Echinoderms[edit]

The earliest generally accepted echinoderm fossils appeared in the Late Atdabanian; unlike modern echinoderms, these early Cambrian echinoderms were not all radially symmetrical.[86] These provide firm data points for the "end" of the explosion, or at least indications that the crown groups of modern phyla were represented.

Burrowing[edit]

Main article: Cambrian substrate revolution

Around the start of the Cambrian (about 539 million years ago), many new types of traces first appear, including well-known vertical burrows such as Diplocraterion and Skolithos, and traces normally attributed to arthropods, such as Cruziana and Rusophycus. The vertical burrows indicate that worm-like animals acquired new behaviours, and possibly new physical capabilities. Some Cambrian trace fossils indicate that their makers possessed hard exoskeletons, although they were not necessarily mineralised.[76] Meiofaunal as well as macrofaunal bilaterians participated in this invasion of infaunal niches.[87]

Burrows provide firm evidence of complex organisms; they are also much more readily preserved than body fossils, to the extent that the absence of trace fossils has been used to imply the genuine absence of large, motile, bottom-dwelling organisms.[citation needed] They provide a further line of evidence to show that the Cambrian explosion

represents a real diversification, and is not a preservational artifact.[88]
Skeletonisation[edit]

The first Ediacaran and lowest Cambrian (Nemakit-Daldynian) skeletal fossils represent tubes and problematic sponge spicules.[89] The oldest sponge spicules are monaxon siliceous, aged around 580 million years ago, known from the Doushantou Formation in China and from deposits of the same age in Mongolia, although the interpretation of these fossils as spicules has been challenged.[90] In the late Ediacaran-lowest Cambrian, numerous tube dwellings of enigmatic organisms appeared. It was organic-walled tubes (e.g. Saarina) and chitinous tubes of the sabelliditids (e.g. Sokoloviina, Sabellidites, Paleolina)[91] [92] that prospered up to the beginning of the Tommotian. The mineralized tubes of Cloudina, Namacalathus, Sinotubulites, and a dozen more of the other organisms from carbonate rocks formed near the end of the Ediacaran period from 549 to 542 million years ago, as well as the triradially symmetrical mineralized tubes of anabaritids (e.g. Anabarites, Cambrotubulus) from uppermost Ediacaran and lower Cambrian.[93] Ediacaran mineralized tubes are often found in carbonates of the stromatolite reefs and thrombolites,[94][95] i.e. they could live in an environment adverse to the majority of animals.

Although they are as hard to classify as most other Ediacaran organisms, they are important in two other ways. First, they are the earliest known calcifying organisms (organisms that built shells from calcium carbonate).[95][96][97] Secondly, these tubes are a device to rise over a substrate and competitors for effective feeding and, to a lesser degree, they serve as armor for protection against predators and adverse conditions of environment. Some Cloudina fossils show small holes in shells. The holes possibly are evidence of boring by predators sufficiently advanced to penetrate shells.[98] A possible "evolutionary arms race" between predators and prey is one of the hypotheses that attempt to explain the Cambrian explosion.[63]

In the lowest Cambrian, the stromatolites were decimated. This allowed animals to begin colonization of warm-water pools with carbonate sedimentation. At first, it was anabaritids and Protohertzina (the fossilized grasping spines of chaetognaths) fossils. Such mineral skeletons as shells, sclerites, thorns, and plates appeared in uppermost Nemakit-Daldynian; they were the earliest species of halkierids, gastropods, hyoliths and other rare organisms. The beginning of the Tommotian has historically been understood to mark an explosive increase of the number and variety of fossils of molluscs, hyoliths, and sponges, along with a rich complex of skeletal

elements   of   unknown   animals,   the
first archaeocyathids, brachiopods, tommotiids, and others.[99][100]
[101][102] Also soft-bodied extant phyla such as comb
jellies,   scalidophorans,   entoproctans,   horseshoe
worms and lobopodians had armored forms.[103] This sudden increase
is partially an artefact of missing strata at the Tommotian type section,
and most of this fauna in fact began to diversify in a series of pulses
through the Nemakit-Daldynian and into the Tommotian.[104]
Some animals may already have had sclerites, thorns, and plates
in the Ediacaran (e.g. Kimberella had hard sclerites, probably
of carbonate), but thin carbonate skeletons cannot be fossilized
in siliciclastic deposits.[105] Older (~750 Ma) fossils indicate that
mineralization long preceded the Cambrian, probably defending small
photosynthetic algae from single-celled eukaryotic predators.[106]
[107]
Burgess Shale type faunas[edit]
Main article: Burgess Shale-type preservation
The Burgess Shale and similar lagerstätten preserve the soft parts of
organisms, which provide a wealth of data to aid in the classification of
enigmatic fossils. It often preserved complete specimens of organisms
only otherwise known from dispersed parts, such as loose scales or
isolated mouthparts. Further, the majority of organisms and taxa in
these horizons are entirely soft-bodied, hence absent from the rest of
the fossil record.[108] Since a large part of the ecosystem is preserved,
the ecology of the community can also be tentatively reconstructed.
[verification needed] However, the assemblages may represent a
"museum": a deep-water ecosystem that is evolutionarily "behind" the
rapidly diversifying fauna of shallower waters.[109]
Because the lagerstätten provide a mode and quality of preservation
that is virtually absent outside of the Cambrian, many organisms
appear completely different from anything known from the
conventional fossil record. This led early workers in the field to attempt
to shoehorn the organisms into extant phyla; the shortcomings of
this approach led later workers to erect a multitude of new phyla to
accommodate all the oddballs. It has since been realised that most
oddballs diverged from lineages before they established the phyla
known today[clarification needed] – slightly different designs, which
were fated to perish rather than flourish into phyla, as their cousin
lineages did.
The preservational mode is rare in the preceding Ediacaran period,
but those assemblages known show no trace of animal life – perhaps

implying a genuine absence of macroscopic metazoans.[110]

Stages[edit]

The early Cambrian interval of diversification lasted for about the next 20[6][7]–25[8][111] million years, and its elevated rates of evolution had ended by the base of Cambrian Series 2, 521 million years ago, coincident with the first trilobites in the fossil record.[112] Different authors define intervals of diversification during the early Cambrian different ways:

Ed Landing recognizes three stages: Stage 1, spanning the Ediacaran-Cambrian boundary, corresponds to a diversification of biomineralizing animals and of deep and complex burrows; Stage 2, corresponding to the radiation of molluscs and stem-group Brachiopods (hyoliths and tommotiids), which apparently arose in intertidal waters; and Stage 3, seeing the Atdabanian diversification of trilobites in deeper waters, but little change in the intertidal realm. [113]

Graham Budd synthesises various schemes to produce a compatible view of the SSF record of the Cambrian explosion, divided slightly differently into four intervals: a "Tube world", lasting from 550 to 536 million years ago, spanning the Ediacaran-Cambrian boundary, dominated by Cloudina, Namacalathus and pseudoconodont-type elements; a "Sclerite world", seeing the rise of halkieriids, tommotiids, and hyoliths, lasting to the end of the Fortunian (c. 525 Ma); a brachiopod world, perhaps corresponding to the as yet unratified Cambrian Stage 2; and Trilobite World, kicking off in Stage 3.[114]

Complementary to the shelly fossil record, trace fossils can be divided into five subdivisions: "Flat world" (late Ediacaran), with traces restricted to the sediment surface; Protreozoic III (after Jensen), with increasing complexity; pedum world, initiated at the base of the Cambrian with the base of the T.pedum zone (see Cambrian#Dating the Cambrian); Rusophycus world, spanning 536 to 521 million years ago and thus corresponding exactly to the periods of Sclerite World and Brachiopod World under the SSF paradigm; and Cruziana world, with an obvious correspondence to Trilobite World. [114]

Validity[edit]

There is strong evidence for species of Cnidaria and Porifera existing in the Ediacaran[115] and possible members of Porifera even before that during the Cryogenian.[116] Bryozoans, once thought to not appear in the fossil record until after the Cambrian, are now known from strata of Cambrian Age 3 from Australia and South China.[117]

The fossil record as Darwin knew it seemed to suggest that the major metazoan groups appeared in a few million years of the early to mid-Cambrian, and even in the 1980s, this still appeared to be the case.[27][28]

However, evidence of Precambrian Metazoa is gradually accumulating. If the Ediacaran Kimberella was a mollusc-like protostome (one of the two main groups of coelomates),[32][70] the protostome and deuterostome lineages must have split significantly before 550 million years ago (deuterostomes are the other main group of coelomates).[118] Even if it is not a protostome, it is widely accepted as a bilaterian.[74][118] Since fossils of rather modern-looking cnidarians (jellyfish-like organisms) have been found in the Doushantuo lagerstätte, the cnidarian and bilaterian lineages must have diverged well over 580 million years ago.[118]

Trace fossils[68] and predatory borings in Cloudina shells provide further evidence of Ediacaran animals.[119] Some fossils from the Doushantuo formation have been interpreted as embryos and one (Vernanimalcula) as a bilaterian coelomate, although these interpretations are not universally accepted.[120][121][122] Earlier still, predatory pressure has acted on stromatolites and acritarchs since around 1,250 million years ago.[63]

Some say that the evolutionary change was accelerated by an order of magnitude,[d] but the presence of Precambrian animals somewhat dampens the "bang" of the explosion; not only was the appearance of animals gradual, but their evolutionary radiation ("diversification") may also not have been as rapid as once thought. Indeed, statistical analysis shows that the Cambrian explosion was no faster than any of the other radiations in animals' history.[e] However, it does seem that some innovations linked to the explosion – such as resistant armour – only evolved once in the animal lineage; this makes a lengthy Precambrian animal lineage harder to defend.[124] Further, the conventional view that all the phyla arose in the Cambrian is flawed; while the phyla may have diversified in this time period, representatives of the crown groups of many phyla do not appear until much later in the Phanerozoic.[13] Further, the mineralised phyla that form the basis of the fossil record may not be representative of other phyla, since most mineralised phyla originated in a benthic setting. The fossil record is consistent with a Cambrian explosion that was limited to the benthos, with pelagic phyla evolving much later.[13]

Ecological complexity among marine animals increased in the Cambrian, as well later in the Ordovician.[12] However, recent research has overthrown the once-popular idea that disparity was exceptionally high throughout the Cambrian, before subsequently decreasing. [125] In fact, disparity remains relatively low throughout the Cambrian, with modern levels of disparity only attained after the early Ordovician radiation.[12]

The diversity of many Cambrian assemblages is similar to today's, [126][84] and at a high (class/phylum) level, diversity is thought by some to have risen relatively smoothly through the Cambrian, stabilizing somewhat in the Ordovician.[127] This interpretation, however, glosses over the astonishing and fundamental pattern of basal polytomy and phylogenetic telescoping at or near the Cambrian boundary, as seen in most major animal lineages.[128] Thus Harry Blackmore Whittington's questions regarding the abrupt nature of the Cambrian explosion remain, and have yet to be satisfactorily answered. [129]

The Cambrian explosion as survivorship bias[edit]

Budd and Mann[130] suggested that the Cambrian explosion was the result of a type of survivorship bias called the "Push of the past". As groups at their origin tend to go extinct, it follows that any long-lived group would have experienced an unusually rapid rate of diversification early on, creating the illusion of a general speed-up in diversification rates. However, rates of diversification could remain at background levels and still generate this sort of effect in the surviving lineages.

Possible causes[edit]

Despite the evidence that moderately complex animals (triploblastic bilaterians) existed before and possibly long before the start of the Cambrian, it seems that the pace of evolution was exceptionally fast in the early Cambrian. Possible explanations for this fall into three broad categories: environmental, developmental, and ecological changes. Any explanation must explain both the timing and magnitude of the explosion.

Changes in the environment[edit]

Increase in oxygen levels[edit]

Earth's earliest atmosphere contained no free oxygen (O_2); the oxygen that animals breathe today, both in the air and dissolved in water, is the product of billions of years of photosynthesis. Cyanobacteria were the first organisms to evolve the ability to photosynthesize, introducing a steady supply of oxygen into the environment.[131] Initially, oxygen levels did not increase substantially in the atmosphere. [132] The oxygen quickly reacted with iron and other minerals in the surrounding rock and ocean water. Once a saturation point was reached for the reactions in rock and water, oxygen was able to exist as a gas in its diatomic form. Oxygen levels in the atmosphere increased substantially afterward.[133] As a general trend, the concentration of oxygen in the atmosphere has risen gradually over about the last 2.5 billion years.[24]

Oxygen levels seem to have a positive correlation with diversity in eukaryotes well before the Cambrian period.[134] The last common ancestor of all extant eukaryotes is thought to have lived around 1.8 billion years ago. Around 800 million years ago, there was a notable increase in the complexity and number of eukaryotes species in the fossil record.[134] Before the spike in diversity, eukaryotes are thought to have lived in highly sulfuric environments. Sulfide interferes with mitochondrial function in aerobic organisms, limiting the amount of oxygen that could be used to drive metabolism. Oceanic sulfide levels decreased around 800 million years ago, which supports the importance of oxygen in eukaryotic diversity.[134] The increased ventilation of the oceans by sponges, which had already evolved and diversified during the Neoproterozoic, has been proposed to have increased the availability of oxygen and powered the Cambrian's rapid diversification of multicellular life.[135][136] Molybdenum isotopes show that increases in biodiversity were strongly correlated with expansion of oxygenated bottom waters in the Early Cambrian, lending support for oxygen as a driver of the Cambrian evolutionary radiation. [137]

The shortage of oxygen might well have prevented the rise of large, complex animals. The amount of oxygen an animal can absorb is largely determined by the area of its oxygen-absorbing surfaces (lungs and gills in the most complex animals; the skin in less complex ones), while the amount needed is determined by its volume, which grows faster than the oxygen-absorbing area if an animal's size increases equally in all directions. An increase in the concentration of oxygen in air or water would increase the size to which an organism could grow without its tissues becoming starved of oxygen. However, members of the Ediacara biota reached metres in length tens of millions of years before the Cambrian explosion.[51] Other metabolic functions may have been inhibited by lack of oxygen, for example the construction of tissue such as collagen, which is required for the construction of complex structures,[138] or the biosynthesis of molecules for the construction of a hard exoskeleton.[139] However, animals were not affected when similar oceanographic conditions occurred in the Phanerozoic;

therefore, some see no forcing role of the oxygen level on evolution.
[140]

Ozone formation[edit]

The amount of ozone (O_3) required to shield Earth from biologically lethal UV radiation, wavelengths from 200 to 300 nanometers (nm), is believed to have been in existence around the Cambrian explosion. [141] The presence of the ozone layer may have enabled the development of complex life and life on land, as opposed to life being restricted to the water.

Snowball Earth[edit]

Main article: Snowball Earth

In the late Neoproterozoic (extending into the early Ediacaran period), the Earth suffered massive glaciations in which most of its surface was covered by ice. This may have caused a mass extinction, creating a genetic bottleneck; the resulting diversification may have given rise to the Ediacara biota, which appears soon after the last "Snowball Earth" episode.[142] However, the snowball episodes occurred a long time before the start of the Cambrian, and it is difficult to see how so much diversity could have been caused by even a series of bottlenecks; [53] the cold periods may even have delayed the evolution of large size organisms.[63] Massive rock erosion caused by glaciers during the "Snowball Earth" may have deposited nutrient-rich sediments into the oceans, setting the stage for the Cambrian explosion.[143]

Increase in the calcium concentration of the Cambrian seawater[edit]

Newer research suggests that volcanically active midocean ridges caused a massive and sudden surge of the calcium concentration in the oceans, making it possible for marine organisms to build skeletons and hard body parts.[144] Alternatively a high influx of ions could have been provided by the widespread erosion that produced Powell's Great Unconformity.[145]

An increase of calcium may also have been caused by erosion of the Transgondwanan Supermountain that existed at the time of the explosion. The roots of the mountain are preserved in present-day East Africa as an orogen.[146]

Developmental explanations[edit]

Further information: Evolutionary developmental biology

A range of theories are based on the concept that minor modifications to animals' development as they grow from embryo to adult may have been able to cause very large changes in the final adult form. The Hox genes, for example, control which organs individual regions of an embryo will develop into. For instance, if a certain Hox gene is expressed, a region will develop into a limb; if a different Hox gene is expressed in that region (a minor change), it could develop into an eye instead (a phenotypically major change).

Such a system allows a large range of disparity to appear from a limited set of genes, but such theories linking this with the explosion struggle to explain why the origin of such a development system should by itself lead to increased diversity or disparity. Evidence of Precambrian metazoans[53] combines with molecular data[147] to show that much of the genetic architecture that could feasibly have played a role in the explosion was already well established by the Cambrian.

This apparent paradox is addressed in a theory that focuses on the physics of development. It is proposed that the emergence of simple multicellular forms provided a changed context and spatial scale in which novel physical processes and effects were mobilized by the products of genes that had previously evolved to serve unicellular functions. Morphological complexity (layers, segments, lumens, appendages) arose, in this view, by self-organization.[148]

Horizontal gene transfer has also been identified as a possible factor in the rapid acquisition of the biochemical capability of biomineralization among organisms during this period, based on evidence that the gene for a critical protein in the process was originally transferred from a bacterium into sponges.[149]

Ecological explanations[edit]

These focus on the interactions between different types of organism. Some of these hypotheses deal with changes in the food chain; some suggest arms races between predators and prey, and others focus on the more general mechanisms of coevolution. Such theories are well suited to explaining why there was a rapid increase in both disparity and diversity, but they do not explain why the "explosion" happened when it did.[53]

End-Ediacaran mass extinction[edit]

Main article: End-Ediacaran extinction

Evidence for such an extinction includes the disappearance from the fossil record of the Ediacara biota and shelly fossils such as Cloudina, and the accompanying perturbation in the δ13C record. It is suspected that several global anoxic events were responsible for the extinction.[150][151]

Mass extinctions are often followed by adaptive radiations as existing clades expand to occupy the ecospace emptied by the extinction. However, once the dust had settled, overall disparity and diversity returned to the pre-extinction level in each of the Phanerozoic extinctions.[53]

Anoxia[edit]

The late Ediacaran oceans appears to have suffered from an anoxia that covered much of the seafloor, which would have given mobile animals with the ability to seek out more oxygen-rich environments an advantage over sessile forms of life.[152]

Increase in sensory and cognitive abilities[edit]

Main article: Evolution of the eye

Andrew Parker has proposed that predator-prey relationships changed dramatically after eyesight evolved. Prior to that time, hunting and evading were both close-range affairs – smell, vibration, and touch were the only senses used. When predators could see their prey from a distance, new defensive strategies were needed. Armor, spines, and similar defenses may also have evolved in response to vision. He further observed that, where animals lose vision in unlighted environments such as caves, diversity of animal forms tends to decrease. [153] Nevertheless, many scientists doubt that vision could have caused the explosion. Eyes may well have evolved long before the start of the Cambrian.[154] It is also difficult to understand why the evolution of eyesight would have caused an explosion, since other senses, such as smell and pressure detection, can detect things at a greater distance in the sea than sight can, but the appearance of these other senses apparently did not cause an evolutionary explosion.[53]

One hypothesis posits that the development of increased cognitive abilities during the Cambrian drove diversity increase. This is evidenced by the fact that the novel ecological lifestyles created during the Cambrian required rapid, regular movement, a feature associated with brain-bearing organisms. The increasing complexity of brains, positively correlated with a greater range of motion and sensory abilities, enabled a wider range of novel ecological modes of life to come into being.[155]

Arms races between predators and prey[edit]

The ability to avoid or recover from predation often makes the difference between life and death, and is therefore one of the strongest components of natural selection. The pressure to adapt is stronger on the prey than on the predator: if the predator fails to win a contest, it loses a meal; if the prey is the loser, it loses its life.[156]

But, there is evidence that predation was rife long before the start of the Cambrian, for example in the increasingly spiny forms of acritarchs, the holes drilled in Cloudina shells, and traces of burrowing to avoid predators. Hence, it is unlikely that the appearance of predation was the trigger for the Cambrian "explosion", although it may well have exhibited a strong influence on the body forms that the "explosion" produced.[63] However, the intensity of predation does appear to have increased dramatically during the Cambrian[157] as new predatory "tactics" (such as shell-crushing) emerged.[158] This rise of predation during the Cambrian was confirmed by the temporal pattern of the median predator ratio at the scale of genus, in fossil communities covering the Cambrian and Ordovician periods, but this pattern is not correlated to diversification rate.[159] This lack of correlation between predator ratio and diversification over the Cambrian and Ordovician suggests that predators did not trigger the large evolutionary radiation of animals during this interval. Thus the role of predators as triggerers of diversification may have been limited to the very beginning of the "Cambrian explosion".[159]

Increase in size and diversity of planktonic animals[edit]

Geochemical evidence strongly indicates that the total mass of plankton has been similar to modern levels since early in the Proterozoic. Before the start of the Cambrian, their corpses and droppings were too small to fall quickly towards the seabed, since their drag was about the same as their weight. This meant they were destroyed by scavengers or by chemical processes before they reached the sea floor.[43]

Mesozooplankton are plankton of a larger size. Early Cambrian specimens filtered microscopic plankton from the seawater. These larger organisms would have produced droppings and ultimately corpses large enough to fall fairly quickly. This provided a new supply of energy and nutrients to the mid-levels and bottoms of the seas, which opened up a new range of possible ways of life. If any of these remains sank uneaten to the sea floor they could be buried; this would have taken some carbon out of circulation, resulting in an increase in the concentration of breathable oxygen in the seas (carbon readily combines with oxygen).[43]

The initial herbivorous mesozooplankton were probably larvae of benthic (seafloor) animals. A larval stage was probably an evolutionary innovation driven by the increasing level of predation at the seafloor during the Ediacaran period.[11][160]

Metazoans have an amazing ability to increase diversity through coevolution.[65] This means that an organism's traits can lead to traits evolving in other organisms; a number of responses are possible, and a different species can potentially emerge from each one.

As a simple example, the evolution of predation may have caused one organism to develop a defence, while another developed motion to flee. This would cause the predator lineage to diverge into two species: one that was good at chasing prey, and another that was good at breaking through defences. Actual coevolution is somewhat more subtle, but, in this fashion, great diversity can arise: three quarters of living species are animals, and most of the rest have formed by coevolution with animals.[65]

Ecosystem engineering[edit]

Evolving organisms inevitably change the environment they evolve in. The Devonian colonization of land had planet-wide consequences for sediment cycling and ocean nutrients, and was likely linked to the Devonian mass extinction. A similar process may have occurred on smaller scales in the oceans, with, for example, the sponges filtering particles from the water and depositing them in the mud in a more digestible form; or burrowing organisms making previously unavailable resources available for other organisms.[161]

Burrowing[edit]

Increases in burrowing changed the seafloor's geochemistry, and led to decreased oxygen in the ocean and increased CO_2 levels in the seas and the atmosphere, resulting in global warming for tens of millions years, and could be responsible for mass extinctions.[162] But as burrowing became established, it allowed an explosion of its own, for as burrowers disturbed the sea floor, they aerated it, mixing oxygen into the toxic muds. This made the bottom sediments more hospitable, and allowed a wider range of organisms to inhabit them – creating new niches and the scope for higher diversity.[88]

Complexity threshold[edit]

The explosion may not have been a significant evolutionary event. It may represent a threshold being crossed: for example a threshold in genetic complexity that allowed a vast range of morphological forms to be employed.[163] This genetic threshold may have a correlation to the amount of oxygen available to organisms. Using oxygen for metabolism produces much more energy than anaerobic processes. Organisms that use more oxygen have the opportunity to produce more complex proteins, providing a template for further evolution.[132] These proteins translate into larger, more complex structures that allow organisms better to adapt to their environments.[164] With the help of oxygen, genes that code for these proteins could contribute to the expression of complex traits more efficiently. Access to a wider range of structures and functions would allow organisms to evolve in different directions, increasing the number of niches that could be inhabited. Furthermore, organisms had the opportunity to become more specialized in their own niches.[164]

Relationship with the Great Ordovician Biodiversification Event[edit]

Main article: Great Ordovician Biodiversification Event

After an extinction at the Cambrian–Ordovician boundary, another radiation occurred, which established the taxa that would dominate the Palaeozoic. This event, known as the Great Ordovician Biodiversification Event (GOBE), has been considered a "follow-up" to the Cambrian explosion.[165] Recent studies have suggested that the Cambrian explosion were not two discrete events but one long evolutionary radiation.[166] Analytical study of the Geobiodiversity Database (GBDB) and Paleobiology Database (PBDB) failed to find a statistical basis for separating the two radiations.[167]

Some researchers have proposed the existence of a biodiversity gap during the Furongian separating the Cambrian explosion and GOBE known as the Furongian Gap.[168] Studies of the Guole Konservat-Lagerstätte and similar fossil sites in South China have instead found the Furongian to instead be a time of rapid biological turnovers though, making the existence of the Furongian Gap highly controversial.[169]

Uniqueness of the early Cambrian biodiversification[edit]

The "Cambrian explosion" can be viewed as two waves of metazoan expansion into empty niches: first, a coevolutionary rise in diversity as animals explored niches on the Ediacaran sea floor, followed by a second expansion in the early Cambrian as they became established in the water column.[65] The rate of diversification seen in the Cambrian phase of the explosion is unparalleled among marine animals: it affected all metazoan clades of which Cambrian fossils have been found. Later radiations, such as those of fish in the Silurian and Devonian periods, involved fewer taxa, mainly with very similar body plans.[24] Although the recovery from the Permian-Triassic extinction started with about as few animal species as the Cambrian explosion, the recovery produced far fewer significantly new types of animals.[170]

Whatever triggered the early Cambrian diversification opened up an exceptionally wide range of previously unavailable ecological niches. When these were all occupied, limited space existed for such wide-ranging diversifications to occur again, because strong competition existed in all niches and incumbents usually had the advantage. If a wide range of empty niches had continued, clades would be able to continue diversifying and become disparate enough for us to recognise them as different phyla; when niches are filled, lineages will continue to resemble one another long after they diverge, as limited opportunity exists for them to change their life-styles and forms.[171]

There were two similar explosions in the evolution of land plants: after a cryptic history beginning about 450 million years ago, land plants underwent a uniquely rapid adaptive radiation during the Devonian period, about 400 million years ago.[24] Furthermore, angiosperms (flowering plants) originated and rapidly diversified during the Cretaceous period. - wiki

LEVERAGE

Leverage - the **exertion** of **<u>force</u>** by means of a lever or an object used in the manner of a **lever,** mechanical advantage gained by using leverage. The power to influence a person or situation to achieve a particular outcome. The ratio of a company's loan capital (debt) to the value of its common stock (equity). To use (something) to maximum advantage.

Force - strength or energy as an attribute of physical action or movement. To make (someone) do something against their will.

Lever - a rigid bar resting on a **pivot**, used to help move a heavy or firmly fixed load with one end when **pressure** is applied to the other. To lift or move with a lever.

Pivot - the central point, pin, or shaft on which a mechanism turns or **oscillates**.

Oscillates - To move or swing back and forth at a regular speed. To waver between **extremes** of opinion, action, or quality. To vary in magnitude or position in a regular manner around a central point. To cause the electric current or voltage running through it to vary in magnitude or position in a regular manner around a central point.

This is the origin of Martial Arts. Yes, Freemasonry, Kemetic Religious Science and Martial Arts is based on Biochemistry & Anatomy.

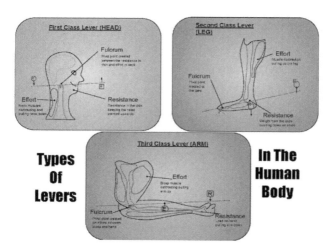

Types Of Levers **In The Human Body**

"Pressure points" and "Joint Locks" are based on knowing anatomy and the design of the body. The body has a linear lever design. Your ankles, knees and elbows are levers.

Your bones are all lever arms.

Your joints are all pivots.

Your blood (through the muscle) provides the power.

Levers are classified by the relative positions of the fulcrum, effort and resistance (or load). It is common to call the input force "effort" and the output force "load" or "resistance". This allows the identification of three classes of levers by the relative locations of the fulcrum, the resistance and the effort:[7]

- Class I – Fulcrum is located between the effort and the resistance: The effort is applied on one side of the fulcrum and the resistance (or load) on the other side. For example, a seesaw, a crowbar, a pair of scissors, a balance scale, a pair of pliers, and a claw hammer (pulling a nail). With the fulcrum in the middle, the lever's mechanical advantage may be greater than, less than, or even equal to 1.

- Class II – Resistance (or load) is located between the effort and the fulcrum: The effort is applied on one side of the resistance and the fulcrum is located on the other side, e.g. a wheelbarrow, a nutcracker, a bottle opener, a wrench, and the brake pedal of a car. Since the load arm is smaller than the effort arm, the lever's mechanical advantage is always greater than 1. It is also called a force multiplier lever.

- Class III – Effort is located between the resistance and the fulcrum: The resistance (or load) is applied on one side of the effort and the fulcrum is located on the other side, e.g. a pair of tweezers, a hammer, a pair of tongs, a fishing rod, and the mandible of a human skull. Since the effort arm is smaller than the load arm, the lever's mechanical advantage is always less than 1. It is also called a speed multiplier lever.

These cases are described by the mnemonic fre 123 where:

the f fulcrum is between r and e for the 1st class lever.

the r resistance is between f and e for the 2nd class lever.

the e effort is between f and r for the 3rd class lever. - wiki

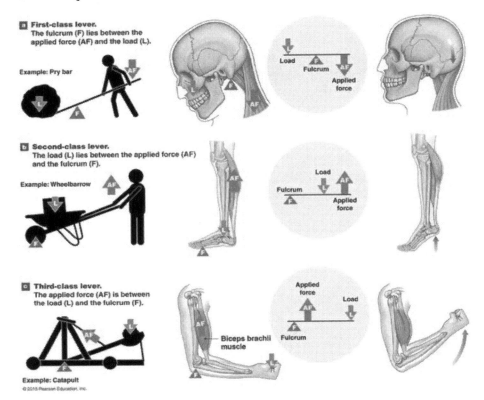

A First-class lever.
The fulcrum (F) lies between the applied force (AF) and the load (L).

Example: Pry bar

B Second-class lever.
The load (L) lies between the applied force (AF) and the fulcrum (F).

Example: Wheelbarrow

C Third-class lever.
The applied force (AF) is between the load (L) and the fulcrum (F).

Example: Catapult
© 2015 Pearson Education, Inc.

The word "lever" entered **English** around AD 1300 from **Old French**: levier. This sprang from the stem of the verb lever, meaning "to raise". The verb, in turn, goes back to **Latin**: levare,[1] itself from the adjective levis, meaning "light" (as in "not heavy"). The word's primary origin is the **Proto-Indo-European** stem legwh-, meaning "light", "easy" or "nimble", among other things. The PIE stem also gave rise to the English word "light".[2] The earliest evidence of the lever mechanism dates back to the **ancient Near East** c. 5000 BC, when it was first used in a simple **balance scale**.[3] In **ancient Egypt** c. 4400 BC, a foot pedal was used for the earliest horizontal frame loom.

[4] In Mesopotamia (modern Iraq) c. 3000 BC, the shadouf, a crane-like device that uses a lever mechanism, was invented.[3] In ancient Egypt, workmen used the lever to move and uplift obelisks weighing more than 100 tons. This is evident from the recesses in the large blocks and the handling bosses which could not be used for any purpose other than for levers.[5]

The earliest remaining writings regarding levers date from the 3rd century BC and were provided by the Greek mathematician Archimedes, who famously stated "Give me a lever long enough and a fulcrum on which to place it, and I shall move the world." - wiki

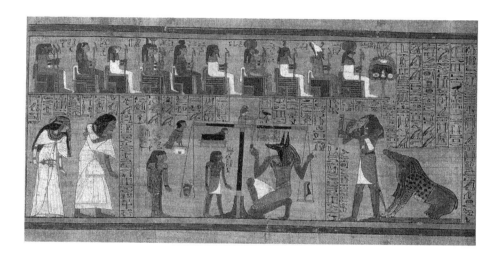

We forget that this is the earliest depiction of a Lever on Earth. We get so lost in the rest of the narrative we forget that this was advanced technology! Very very advanced technology! The scale is a whole entire science unto itself!!! We are going to dig into this scene but we have to begin here. The blueprint of the body is the Lever! Our body is built as arms, pivots and the infinite ability to generate force.

We are designed as the perfect levers, think about it, as we use the levers (exercise) it strengthens our ability to generate force, to use the lever. Using the levers, our limbs, requires muscle which requires blood, which requires oxygen. The more you use each lever system, the system is strengthened! If you stop using any of them, they are designed to atrophy so that more resources can be directed to the levers you are using. If you want **BALANCED STRENGTH**, you must use them all.

This is blatant, the Heart and the Feather on the scale!!! I have been telling these "Scholars" that this is about balance between Electricity (feather) and Magnetism (heart). The Soul (electricity) and the Spirit (magnetism).

Cardiac torsion and electromagnetic fields: the cardiac bioinformation hypothesis

Katharine O Burleson 1, Gary E Schwartz
Affiliations expand

  • PMID: 15823696 DOI: 10.1016/j.mehy.2004.12.023

Abstract

Although in physiology the heart is often referred to as a simple piston pump, there are in fact two additional features that are integral to cardiac physiology and function. First, the heart as it contracts in systole, also rotates and produces torsion due to the structure of the myocardium. Second, the heart produces a significant electromagnetic field with each contraction due to the coordinated depolarization of myocytes producing a current flow. Unlike the electrocardiogram, the magnetic field is not limited to volume conduction and extends outside the body. The therapeutic potential for interaction of this cardioelectromagnetic field both within and outside the body is largely unexplored. It is our hypothesis that the heart functions as a generator of bioinformation that is central to normative functioning of body. The source of this bioinformation is based on: (1) vortex blood flow in the left ventricle; (2) a cardiac electromagnetic field and both; (3) heart sounds; and (4) pulse pressure which produce frequency and amplitude information. Thus, there is a multidimensional role for the heart in physiology and biopsychosocial dynamics. Recognition of these cardiac properties may result in significant implications for new therapies for cardiovascular disease based on increasing cardiac energy efficiency (coherence) and bioinformation from the cardioelectromagnetic field. Research studies to test this hypothesis are suggested.

We won't do a big "to do" about the Heart here, we have discussed the heart quite a bit in many of the books. Please read and/or reread them all. This book is for better understanding of the Feather. In the L'Goat book pages 419-431 we examined a Article on the Traditional Chinese Meridians and the Fascia. The results were very different than what meridian supporters would've hoped for and vastly different than what skeptics hoped for.

In this book we are going to look at the Fascia from it's introduction in the Weighing of the Heart Ceremony and what modern science tells us, creating a comparative analysis to extrapolate what we need to know to be healthy. To put it plainly "How to Wash our A$$" LOL....

If you do not hydrate and eat a certain way, combined with routine exercise, YOU HAVE NOT WASH YOUR BOOTY!!! Imagine some people go decades without washing!!!

This is the reason that there is a secret tradition of Bone Marrow Washing. It is about directing energy inwards through exercise and how the Fascia behave. How the Heart powers the movement of the scales, via your Feathers. This is probably the biggest paradigm shift from one of my discoveries thus far! We are made out of feathers?

The brain is even dependent maybe more than any other structure in the body on these Feathers! Which makes the depiction of the "Bird Brain" so insane and miraculous. I don't mean a actual bird brain, I mean the Vault of Heaven. The depiction of the Heru Falcon as the Midbrain!

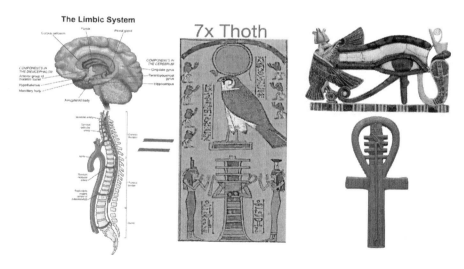

These ancients depictions of Scientific Religious Worship are so epically Rich in Science! Science that we need too, because we are suffering. We are particularly suffering from Mental and Brain decay.

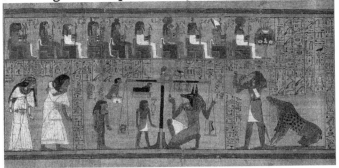

The Scale in the weighing of the Heart Ceremony clearly delineates a solid working and understanding of Levers. Placing the Heart and the Feather on the scale, takes the technology of the scale to even greater depths!

The Fascia carry the waves of the heart to every corner of the body. This is remarkable.

Let's look at this a different way, as humans our Brain gives us leverage over the rest of creation. In the Bible could the term dominion be better translated as leverage? We detailed in the Eye of Heru book aka You got some Nerve book, the advantages our spine give us over "primates", we detailed the differences in our muscle and mitochondria etc…

This is leverage. We dominate with our infinite ability to create and use leverage against or for, ourselves and the rest of the living creatures on this planet. The lever is our physical and mental blueprint it's truly phenomenal. There is no creation of scales without the understanding of leverage. A scale literally measures the leverage of one thing over the other. That's a basic Lever Scale as shown at the center of the weighing of the heart ceremony.

Technology is that concept on steroids!

Vehicles (traveling tools) give us leverage to travel different terrains faster and more securely.

Weapons (fighting/hunting tools) multiply our killing force.

Computers (thinking tools) multiply our ability to process and store information.

Workout equipment (lever tools) multiply our ability to build and store power.

This is all leverage, I hope you see what I am sharing.

Birds of a Feather all flock together!

SINOVIAL FLUID

Hyaluronic Acid - Hyaluronic acid is a natural substance found in the fluids in the eyes and joints. It acts as a cushion and lubricant in the joints and other tissues.

Synovial fluid - joint fluid, is a thick liquid located between your joints. The fluid cushions the ends of bones and reduces friction when you move your joints.

*See the problem there? Most people have never heard of these terms and we have goofballs online seeking to take advantage of the fact people don't know this information. These goofballs use the two terms interchangeably! Hyaluronic Acid goes in the Synovial Fluid, got it? If not don't worry you know we have some articles to add extra clarity for you lol... Lets look at the nutrition (Purple Phaze & Ocean Steak build the joints)...

Hyaluronic acid (HA) is a linear glycosaminoglycan (GAG), an anionic, gel-like, polymer, found in the extracellular matrix of epithelial and connective tissues of vertebrates. It is part of a family of structurally complex, linear, anionic polysaccharides.[7] The carboxylate groups present in the molecule make it negatively charged, therefore allowing for successful binding to water, and making it valuable to cosmetic and pharmaceutical products.[47]

HA consists of repeating β4-glucuronic acid (GlcUA)-β3-N-acetylglucosamine (GlcNAc) disaccharides, and is synthesized by hyaluronan synthases (HAS), a class of integral membrane proteins that produce the well-defined, uniform chain lengths characteristic to HA.[47] There are three existing types of HASs in vertebrates: HAS1, HAS2, HAS3; each of these contribute to elongation of the HA polymer.[7] For an HA capsule to be created, this enzyme must be present because it polymerizes UDP-sugar precursors into HA. HA precursors are synthesized by first phosphorylating glucose by hexokinase, yielding glucose-6-phosphate, which is the main HA precursor.[48] **Then, two routes are taken to synthesize UDP-n-acetylglucosamine and UDP-glucuronic acid which both react to form HA.**

Glucose-6-phosphate gets converted to either fructose-6-phosphate with hasE (phosphoglucoisomerase), or glucose-1-phosphate using pgm (α -phosphoglucomutase), where those both undergo different sets of reactions.[48]

UDP-glucuronic acid and UDP-n-acetylglucosamine get bound together to form HA via hasA (HA synthase).[47]

Precursor 1: Synthesis of UDP-Glucuronic Acid
Synthesis of UDP-glucuronic acid[edit]

UDP-glucuronic acid is formed from hasC (UDP-glucose pyrophosphorylase) converting glucose-1-P into UDP-glucose, which then reacts with hasB (UDP-glucose dehydrogenase) to form UDP-glucuronic acid.[47]

Precursor 2: Synthesis of UDP-N-Acetylglucosamine
Synthesis of N-acetyl glucosamine[edit]

The path forward from fructose-6-P utilizes glmS (amidotransferase) to form glucosamine-6-P. Then, glmM (Mutase) reacts with this product to form glucosamine-1-P. hasD (acetyltransferase) converts this into n-acetylglucosamine-1-P, and finally, hasD (pyrophosphorylase) converts this product into UDP-n-acetylglucosamine.[48]

Final step of HA Synthesis
Final step: Two disaccharides form hyaluronic acid[edit]

UDP-glucuronic acid and UDP-n-acetylglucosamine get bound together to form HA via hasA (HA synthase), completing the synthesis.

Synovial tissue is sterile and composed of vascularized connective tissue that lacks a basement membrane. Two cell types (type A and type B) are present: Type A is derived from blood monocytes, and it removes the wear-and-tear debris from the synovial fluid. Type B produces hyaluronan. **Synovial fluid** is made of **hyaluronic acid and lubricin**, **proteinases, and collagenases**. Synovial fluid exhibits non-Newtonian flow characteristics; the viscosity coefficient is not a constant and the fluid is not linearly viscous. Synovial fluid has thixotropic characteristics; under conditions of sudden increase in pressure as in some kind of mechanical shock, its viscosity suddenly increases.[11] Normal synovial fluid contains 3–4 mg/ml hyaluronan (hyaluronic acid), [12] a polymer of disaccharides composed of D-glucuronic acid and D-N-acetylglucosamine joined by alternating beta-1,4 and beta-1,3 glycosidic bonds.[13][unreliable medical source?] Hyaluronan is synthesized by the synovial membrane and secreted into the joint cavity to increase the viscosity and elasticity of articular cartilages and to lubricate the surfaces between synovium and cartilage.[14] [unreliable medical source?]

Synovial fluid contains lubricin (also known as PRG4) as a second lubricating component, secreted by synovial fibroblasts.[15] Chiefly, it is responsible for so-called boundary-layer lubrication, which reduces friction between opposing surfaces of cartilage. There also is some evidence that it helps regulate synovial cell growth.[16]

It also contains phagocytic cells that remove microbes and the debris that results from normal wear and tear in the joint.

Lubricin shares many properties with other members of the mucin family and similarly plays important roles in protecting cartilage surface from protein deposition and cell adhesion, in inhibiting synovial cell overgrowth, and in preventing cartilage-cartilage adhesion.

Birds of a Feather all flock together!

The blueprint is the blueprint. The toes, ankles, knees, hips, fingers, wrists, elbows & neck are all types of levers!

Let's explore the knee so we can get some understanding on all of the joints via the knee. All joints work basically the same. The knee is the biggest problem area because it is the most vulnerable to the golden rule of Hormesis Training. The body works based on applied pressure and perpetual movement, the base of the body is piezoelectric.

Medial Collateral Ligament - The MCL spans the distance from the end of the femur (thigh bone) to the top of the tibia (shin bone) and is on the inner side of the knee joint.

Posterior Cruciate Ligament - It works as a counterpart to the anterior cruciate ligament (ACL). It connects the posterior intercondylar area of the tibia to the medial condyle of the femur. This configuration allows the PCL to resist forces pushing the tibia posteriorly relative to the femur.

The PCL and ACL are intracapsular ligaments because they lie deep within the knee joint. **They are both isolated from the fluid-filled**

synovial cavity, with the synovial membrane wrapped around them. The PCL gets its name by attaching to the posterior portion of the tibia.

Lateral Collateral Ligament - is an extrinsic ligament of the knee located on the lateral side of the knee. Its superior attachment is at the lateral epicondyle of the femur (superoposterior to the popliteal groove); its inferior attachment is at the lateral aspect of the head of fibula (anterior to the apex). The LCL is not fused with the joint capsule. Inferiorly, the LCL splits the tendon of insertion of the biceps femoris muscle.

Anterior Cruciate Ligament - one of the strong bands of tissue that help connect your thigh bone (femur) to your shinbone (tibia). ACL injuries most commonly occur during sports that involve sudden stops or changes in direction, jumping and landing — such as soccer, basketball, football and downhill skiing.

Zinc

Copper

Vitamin C

Vitamin E

Vitamin D

Allium

Lysine

Proline

Glycine

Hydroxyproline

Omega 3s

Glucosamine

We go into much moor detail in the God = Knowledge book!! Please read and reread that book.

Glucosamine-chondroitin sulphate accelerates tendon-to-bone healing in rabbits

Anil Taşkesen 1, Baybars Ataoğlu, Mustafa Özer, İsmail Demirkale, Sacit Turanli
Affiliations expand

· PMID: 26165711 DOI: 10.5606/ehc.2015.17

Abstract

Objectives: This study aims to investigate the contribution of glucosamine-chondroitin sulphate (GlcN-CS) to the healing of tendons within the bone tunnel.

Materials and methods: Tendon-to-bone healing was investigated in 28 New Zealand rabbits by re-attaching the extensor digitorum longus tendon into bone tunnel which was created in the proximal tibia. Rabbits were separated into two groups as treatment and control groups. Treatment group (n=14) received 210-250 mg/kg/day glucosamine sulphate and 170-200 mg/kg/day chondroitin sulphate, whereas control group (n=14) received equivalent dose of vehicle. Treatment and control groups were compared at sixth and 12th week after the procedure according to histological and biomechanical analysis. Yamakado scoring system was used to evaluate the histological changes.

Results: According to histological analysis, scores were significantly higher at both sixth and 12th week evaluations in the treatment group (p=0.029). Although not statistically significant, the ultimate pullout strength was higher in the treatment group at the 12th week evaluation (35.3 N/mm2 vs. 24.3 N/mm2) (p>0.05). However, stripping occurred at the muscle-tendon junction in the treatment group whereas tendons stripped from the bone tunnels in the control group. While no tendons in the treatment group stripped from the bone tunnels, we observed at sixth and 12th week evaluations that tendons in the control group stripped from the tunnels.

Conclusion: Glucosamine-chondroitin sulphate treatment enhances tendon-to-bone healing by increasing hyaline cartilage formation and decreasing formation of capillary vessels.

Glucosamine ($C_6H_{13}NO_5$) is an amino sugar and a prominent precursor in the biochemical synthesis of glycosylated proteins and lipids. Glucosamine is part of the structure of two polysaccharides, chitosan and chitin. Glucosamine is one of the most abundant monosaccharides.[2] Produced commercially by the hydrolysis of shellfish exoskeletons or, less commonly, by fermentation of a grain such as corn or wheat, glucosamine has many names depending on country.

*We have particular herbs in the Bitters & Purple Phaze to promote the growth of Villi & Glycoproteins!!! The BleuMagick Gel is the ultimate level in joint nutrition with the Bitters & Purple Phaze!!!

Birds of a Feather...

The way this work is similar to the lungs, the lungs function like a balloon with fine holes in them. The magic is the balloons must filled with air and at the same time, allow the oxygen to seep out at a steady rate. The joints are similar balloons but only these are for thicker gel than water.

The body exerts a incredible amount of force on the knees and ankle. The achilles tendon is a runner up to the ligaments in the knees. The bones are designed to float on top of the Gels in the joint capsule. The tendons and ligaments help to stabilize these bones and the weight they carry. The pivot to manage the load and the force is Gel!!!

Go get that BleuMagick Gel now!!!

The Gel creates **HydroDynamic Pressure** inside the joint. The key is to produce Synovial Fluid at a rate equal to its leakage, that's the cycle. The recipe for success is pressure + ingredients = production of the right structures. If you are not using these structures and playing the pressure... Why would your body use resources to build them?

Pain is the healing signal. You can not seek to constantly avoid pain and have the healing you want! If you use knee braces and ankle braces as fashion just know you are weakening the ligaments and tendons!

Moving the joints (exercise) creates the leakage and also the mechanism that drives regeneration at the same time, balance.

No movement or little movement - causes reduced gel in the joints.

Reduced gel in the joints causes pain and discomfort from movement.

Pain and discomfort from movement, prevent movement and increase the desire for "pain killers". This is usually the Excuse Factory engine, my knees aint what they used to be... No its you buddy!

You started working and riding in that car and it was over. Cars kill your joints!!! You can keep a minimum amount of pressure on your joints by walking!!!

*Doing sissy squats allows your knees to build the structures back out in the knee and re-inflate the joints. Now think about sitting and eating all the time, you damn near get up heavier than every time you sit down! *Doing sets of front foot raises on your heels alternating with sets of heel raises on your toes, works all the muscles in the feet!

This is how you send the blood into the feet, **<u>cleaning the kidneys</u>**!

Each time the blood leaves the kidneys that stimulates the kidneys to produce EPO.

THE APRON PART 2

The abdomen functions like a huge complex joint. The fascia that fills the body is full of a variety of Gels.

The same way feather attract electrons to them to create electricity out of the air, our collagen does the same thing internally.

Bowing is a great exercise, it's the opposite to leg lifts. We need steady pressure on the abdomen to keep the proper levels of Hydration, Momatomix is the key to advanced Hydration!!!

Yes not only are there particular nutrients required for Hydration (beyond electrolytes) but hormesis training is required!

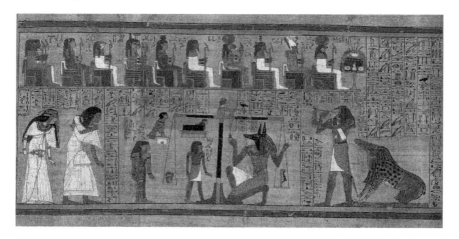

VISCERAL BELLY FAT IS THE MOST DANGEROUS! PARTICULARLY FOR LATINO, BROWN AND BLACK PEOPLE! Your body is not historically designed for it, and we live in a steady temperature! Taking cold baths and showers is cool but its a bandaid. Lets go a step further, the cytokines produced by this type of abdomen fat SHUT DOWN YOUR PIGMENT ESPECIALLY MELANIN! Think about this you Neurons in the heart, and even worse Neurons all through out the gut!!! 500 million to 1 billion Neurons in the digestive system is the current numbers! Enteric Dopaminergic Neurons would be damaged more than any other set of Enteric Neurons/Nerves.

Fat is not completely neutral as we discussed in the You got some Nerve book... First in, last out is the philosophy. Polar Haplotypes have a preference for visceral fat as insulation for organs (triggered by Vitamins D and K), Equatorial Haplotypes have a subcutaneous preference which complicates things a bit... The fat soluble vitamins are still crucial to shedding fat no matter what! This is why we have a superior Banana Oil product that I consume orally and so does my children! Its great for natural vitamin A and E!!!

Dr. W.H. Sheldon in the 1940s based fat storage and muscle tone on the 3 layers of embryonic skin. The Endoderm-Endomorph, the Mesoderm-Mesomorph and the Ectoderm-Ectomorph. His original theory was much more coherent than what it has devolved into over the years. It is now just a tool mass marketing campaigns, by campaigners that don't even understand the roots of the theory.

There is a simple level to it where we can say these cells come from these stem cells, only life isn't that simple. In order to make organs and organ systems cell migrate and not only that different cells build together. Prime example in the abdomen the endoderm cells make the digestive tube but the mesoderm cells surround that tube to build it's peristaltic muscle. Just for example lets look at this VERY SHORT LIST from wiki to get a idea of these cell lines...

This is a list of cells in humans derived from the three embryonic germ layers – ectoderm, mesoderm, and endoderm.

Cells derived from ectoderm[edit]

Surface ectoderm[edit]

Skin[edit]

- Trichocyte
- Keratinocyte

Anterior pituitary[edit]

- Gonadotrope
- Corticotrope
- Thyrotrope
- Somatotrope
- Lactotroph

Tooth enamel[edit]

- Ameloblast

Neural crest[edit]

Peripheral nervous system[edit]

- Neuron
- Glia
  - Schwann cell
  - Satellite glial cell

Neuroendocrine system[edit]

- Chromaffin cell
- Glomus cell

Skin[edit]

- Melanocyte
  - Nevus cell
- Merkel cell

Teeth[edit]

- Odontoblast
- Cementoblast

Eyes[edit]

- Corneal keratocyte

Neural tube[edit]

Central nervous system[edit]

- Neuron
- Glia
  - Astrocyte
  - Ependymocytes
  - Muller glia (retina)
  - Oligodendrocyte
  - Oligodendrocyte progenitor cell
  - Pituicyte (posterior pituitary)

Pineal gland[edit]

- Pinealocyte

Cells derived from mesoderm[edit]

Paraxial mesoderm[edit]

Mesenchymal stem cell[edit]

Osteochondroprogenitor cell[edit]

- Bone (Osteoblast → Osteocyte)
- Cartilage (Chondroblast → Chondrocyte)

Myofibroblast[edit]

- Fat
  - Lipoblast → Adipocyte
- Muscle
  - Myoblast → Myocyte
  - Myosatellite cell
  - Tendon cell
  - Cardiac muscle cell
- Other
  - Fibroblast → Fibrocyte

Other[edit]

- Digestive system
  - Interstitial cell of Cajal

Intermediate mesoderm[edit]

Renal stem cell[edit]

- Angioblast → Endothelial cell
- Mesangial cell

- ○ Intraglomerular
- ○ Extraglomerular
- · Juxtaglomerular cell
- · Macula densa cell
- · Stromal cell → Interstitial cell → Telocytes
- · Simple epithelial cell → Podocyte
- · Kidney proximal tubule brush border cell

Reproductive system[edit]

- · Sertoli cell
- · Leydig cell
- · Granulosa cell
- · Peg cell
- · Germ cells (which migrate here primordially)
  - ○ spermatozoon
  - ○ ovum

Lateral plate mesoderm[edit]

Hematopoietic stem cell[edit]

- · Lymphoid
  - ○ Lymphoblast
  - ○ see lymphocytes
- · Myeloid
  - ○ CFU-GEMM
  - ○ see myeloid cells

Circulatory system[edit]

- · Endothelial progenitor cell
- · Endothelial colony forming cell
- · Endothelial stem cell
- · Angioblast/Mesoangioblast
- · Pericyte
- · Mural cell

Body cavities[edit]

- · Mesothelial cell

Cells derived from endoderm

Foregut[edit]

Respiratory system[edit]

- · Pneumocyte
  - ○ Type I cell

- ○ Type II cell
- Club cell
- Goblet cell
- Pulmonary neuroendocrine cell[1]

Digestive system[edit]

Stomach[edit]

- Enteroendocrine cell
  - ○ G cell
  - ○ Delta cell
  - ○ Enterochromaffin-like cell
- Gastric chief cell
- Parietal cell
- Foveolar cell

Intestine[edit]

- Enteroendocrine cell
  - ○ Gastric inhibitory polypeptide
  - ○ S cell
  - ○ Delta cell
  - ○ Cholecystokinin
  - ○ Enterochromaffin cell
- Goblet cell
- Paneth cell
- Tuft cell
- Enterocyte
  - ○ Microfold cell

Liver[edit]

- Hepatocyte
- Hepatic stellate cell

Gallbladder[edit]

- Cholecystocyte

Exocrine component of pancreas[edit]

- Centroacinar cell
- Pancreatic stellate cell

Islets of Langerhans[edit]

- alpha cell
- beta cell
- delta cell
- PP cell (F cell, gamma cell)

- epsilon cell

Pharyngeal pouch[edit]

- Thyroid gland
  - Follicular cell
  - Parafollicular cell[2]
- Parathyroid gland
  - Parathyroid chief cell
  - Oxyphil cell

Hindgut/cloaca[edit]

- Urothelial cell

There is nobody on earth who is developed by only endoderm or mesoderm cells! What Dr. Sheldon did not know in the 1940s, nor could Dr. Conrad Waddington… was where the science of epigenetics was growing. Conrad may have had the ideas of the potential but honestly Dr. Sheldon may not even have been aware of epigenetics then.

The concept of these body types is actually a combination of two things 1) Haplotypes & 2) the lifestyle of the parents. Those are the two things that contribute to the physical potential in a child. Then we have the inclination, and opportunity of the child early on, to develop habits that reinforce those natural traits. I child born tall may not be exposed to sports until waaaay after his formative years, he may just be a tall chess player or computer programmer.

The body types are not fake because we can clearly see them but they are not endo, meso or ecto based lol… We store fat and build muscle based on our Haplotypes and Genetic Library! We also know now that we can change our gene expression. In the Gold book we give that outline for microRNA influences for a reason! Nutrition and exercise is the blue print to make your own changes! Rewrite your AlgaRhythm!

Somatotype is a theory proposed in the 1940s by the American psychologist William Herbert Sheldon to categorize the human physique according to the relative contribution of three fundamental elements which he termed somatotypes, classified by him as ectomorphic, mesomorphic, and endomorphic. He created these terms borrowing from the three germ layers of embryonic development: The endoderm, (which develops into the digestive tract), the mesoderm, (which becomes muscle, heart, and blood vessels) and the ectoderm (which forms the skin and nervous system).[1] Later variations of these categories, developed by his original research assistant Barbara Heath, and later by Lindsay Carter and Rob Rempel, are used by academics today.[2][3]

Constitutional psychology is a theory developed by Sheldon in the 1940s, which attempted to associate his somatotype classifications with human temperament types.[4][5] The foundation of these ideas originated with Francis Galton and eugenics.[2] Sheldon and Earnest Hooton were seen as leaders of a school of thought, popular in anthropology at the time, which held that the size and shape of a person's body indicated intelligence, moral worth and future achievement.[2]

In his 1954 book, Atlas of Men, Sheldon categorized all possible body types according to a scale ranging from 1 to 7 for each of the three somatotypes, where the pure endomorph is 7–1–1, the pure mesomorph 1–7–1 and the pure ectomorph scores 1–1–7.[6][7][8] From type number, an individual's mental characteristics could supposedly be predicted.[7] In a late version of a pseudoscientific thread within criminology in which criminality is claimed to be an innate characteristic that can be recognized through particular physiognomic markers (as in Cesare Lombroso's theory of phrenology), Sheldon contended that criminals tended to be 'mesomorphic'.[9] The system of somatotyping is still in use in the field of physical education.[10]

The three types[edit]

Comparison of Sheldon's body types
Sheldon's "somatotypes" and their associated physical and psychological traits were characterized as follows:

Somatotype	Physical traits	Psychological traits	Notes
Ectomorphic	characterized as skinny, weak, and usually tall with low testosterone levels	described as intelligent, gentle and calm, but self-conscious, introverted and anxious.	[3][6][8][12]
Mesomorphic	characterized as naturally hard and strong, with even weight distribution, muscular, thick-	described as competitive, extroverted, and tough.	[3][6][8]

54

	skinned, and as having good posture with narrow waist		
Endomorphic	characterized as fat, usually short, and having difficulty losing weight	described as outgoing, friendly, happy and laid-back, but also lazy and selfish	[3][6][8]

Stereotyping[edit]

There may be some evidence that different physiques carry cultural stereotypes, as some cultures are more prone to certain physiques. According to one study endomorphs are likely to be perceived as slow, sloppy, and lazy. Mesomorphs, in contrast, are typically stereotyped as popular and hardworking, whereas ectomorphs are often viewed as intelligent yet fearful.[13]

Heath–Carter formula[edit]

Sheldon's physical taxonomy is still in use, particularly the Heath–Carter variant of the methodology.[14] This formulaic approach utilises an individual's weight (kg), height (cm), upper arm circumference (cm), maximal calf circumference (cm), femur breadth (cm), humerus breadth (cm), triceps skinfold (mm), subscapular skinfold (mm), supraspinal skinfold (mm), and medial calf skinfold (mm), and remains popular in anthropomorphic research, according to Rempel: "with modifications by Parnell in the late 1950s, and by Heath and Carter in the mid 1960s somatotype has continued to be the best single qualifier of total body shape".[15]

This variant utilizes the following series of equations to assess a subject's traits against each of the three somatotypes, each assessed on a seven-point scale, with 0 indicating no correlation and 7 indicating a very strong correlation:

where:

- Ectomorphy : Calculate the subject's **Ponderal Index**:
  - If ,
  - If ,
  - If ,

This numerical approach has gone on to be incorporated in the current **sports science** and **physical education** curriculums of numerous institutions, ranging from the UK's secondary level GCSE curriculums (14- to 16-year-olds), the Indian UPSC Civil Service exams, to MSc programs worldwide, and has been utilized in numerous

academic papers, including:
- Rowing athletes[16]
- Tennis athletes[17]
- Judo athletes[18]
- Volleyball athletes[19]
- Gymnasts[20][21]
- Soccer athletes[22]
- Triathletes[23]
- Han people[24]
- Persons with diabetes[25][26]
- Taekwondo athletes[27]
- Persons with eating disorders[28]
- Dragon boat participants[29]

Criticism[edit]

"The Varieties of Human Physique" by Sheldon et al (1940) classified body types into 3 categories using data processes that would not be accepted by researchers today.[30] Sheldon's ideas that body type was an indicator of temperament, moral character or potential – while popular in an atmosphere accepting of the theories of eugenics – were later disputed.[2][31]

A key criticism of Sheldon's constitutional theory is that it was not a theory at all but a general assumption of continuity between structure and behavior and a set of descriptive concepts to measure physique and behavior in a scaled manner.[3] His use of thousands of photographs of naked Ivy League undergraduates, obtained without explicit consent from a pre-existing program evaluating student posture, has been strongly criticized.[2][32]

While popular in the 1950s,[32] Sheldon's claims have since been dismissed as "quackery".[3][4][33][34][35] Barbara Honeyman Heath, who was Sheldon's main assistant in compiling Atlas of Men, accused him of falsifying the data he used in writing the book. - wiki

Here is the cheat code to Fat burning beyond what we have in Melanin vs Diabetes book 3 the Fiscal Edition, book 4 the Carbon Edition, the Gold Book etc...

Perpetual Motion - The combination of constant activity (physical and mental), this is real activity that gives you a sore feeling in the body, or mental fatigue from abstract study.

Biochemistry and Anatomy are definitely qualified as abstract study!!!

Constantly moving the Blood into and out of the core, consuming loads of gels and gel building nutrients (AmericanHealer.Website)... This is why we practice the LAW of 60 in 60! Its not just 60 pushups or 60 reps in 60 seconds, it's 60 seconds of exercise per hour, on top of your workouts!!! The following are all or at least most of the muscle in your "6 pack", in fact you should see immediately that its much more complicated to build a solid core than a 3 week routine or quick detox!!! There are more than 6 muscle groups and all of these muscle groups have fat and gunk on them!

Sugars, Bio Films, Fat, oh my!

PECTORALIS MAJOR BLENDS INTO THE UPPER RECTUS ABDOMINIS
QUADRATUS LUMBORUM
INTERNAL & EXTERNAL INTERCOSTAL
SUBCOSTAL
TRANSVERSUS THORACIS
TRANSVERSUS ABDOMINIS
PYRAMIDALIS
CREMASTER
INTERNAL OBLIQUE
GREATER OMENTUM (the Apron)
SERRATUS ANTERIOR
LATISSIMUS DORSI
LINEA ALBA
EXTERNAL OBLIQUE APONEUROSIS
EXTERNAL OBLIQUE
RECTUS SHEATH
ILIACUS
PSOAS MAJOR

All of these muscles support one another, overall the majority of the abs are slow twitch (40%-60%), that means designed for high volume. Abs shouldn't be treated like your trying to win Mr. Olympia, high volume is the key.

Sedentary does soften your body and feminize your look, boobs and fat are good for moms and soon to be moms. If you are not in either of those two categories KNOCK IT OFF! Get going! Estrogen will kill you! Fellas you are losing your Y chromosomes from lack of movements, your losing your penis function!!! This means this call out about estrogen storage is to everyone over 30 years old!!! Get rid of the fat!!!

Excess belly fat inhibits the Mesentery organs from their jobs!

Mesentery is a sheet-like structure that encloses the intestine and attaches it to the posterior part of the abdominal wall. The mesentery organs builds collagen and vessels!!!

Fascia is mostly of water with proteins and glycoproteins (Gel). Fascia is made up of 70 percent water which is why hydration is part of the detox protocol. Collagen and elastin provide structure and flexibility to the fascia. Glycoproteins hold the water in the fascial system to keep it supple.

Caffeine or anything that dehydrates the body forces those fascia sheets to stick to each other. This is the perfect environment for biofilms and they become almost impossible to get rid of! Biofilms are little sticky strips that Bacteria live on, each bacteria can host a unlimited number of virus in, see the problem?

Glycoproteins or more specifically proteoglycans are sugary proteins (glycosylated).

Proteoglycans are proteins[1] that are heavily glycosylated. The basic proteoglycan unit consists of a "core protein" with one or more covalently attached glycosaminoglycan (GAG) chain(s). [2] The point of attachment is a serine (Ser) residue to which the glycosaminoglycan is joined through a tetrasaccharide bridge (e.g. chondroitin sulfate-GlcA-Gal-Gal-Xyl-PROTEIN). The Ser residue is generally in the sequence -Ser-Gly-X-Gly- (where X can be any amino acid residue but proline), although not every protein with this sequence has an attached glycosaminoglycan. The chains are long, linear carbohydrate polymers that are negatively charged under physiological conditions due to the occurrence of sulfate and uronic acid groups. Proteoglycans occur in connective tissue. - WIKI

WE ARE STAR FISH

This ultimately becomes a water discussion as usual with me... lol

Interstitial Fluid, Lymph, Blood Plasma, Cytosol, CSF...

In the Fascia you have water that is stored as gel, water becoming gel and water that was gel (becoming something else). The gels are bound via glycosaminoglycans (Mucous shout out to Sebi). This conversion and flow of water is crucial to clean all of your insides!!! You need more than herbs!!! You need more than creatine!!! The Feathers of you wings hold structured water, negatively charged, ready to go!!!

This is the Bleu Magick of the Fascia, you are one big Gel, one big Bleu Magick! There is no greater supplement for Gel than our Gel, many have tried to duplicate the formula but they just don't know enough about the body and plants to do it!

Here is the rub, people that don't exercise and sweat have filthy insides no matter how well they eat or bathe!!! They don't know how to wash they a$$!!! When you exercise you literally squeeze out the old water and clean them feathers! This flushes old water and then soaks up fresh water! This needs to be soaked up via the small intestines soooooo.... The bacteria become crucial....

Who knew that wheat could be food for your joints and ligaments? The Egyptians lol...

They gave us Martial Arts Bread, Beer and Bitters!!!

Now we just gotta do the work, stretching and exercising, flush old water and pull in fresh water, if there is fresh water available right?

Each exercise targets specific muscle groups, each muscle group is going to clean the fascia it is attached to. The dirty water will drain into the lymphatic system **A BIG REASON THE MOMATOMIX IS SO CRUCIAL IN OUR DAILY DIETS**!!! The liver and spleen do their jobs as cleaners providing that you are taking care of them as well... Your circulatory system will circulate new fluids.... Viola! Your insides are getting clean and the more consistently your clean your tissues the deeper the clean gets... It make take years to remove biofilms and completely rejuvenate your body but you literally can just get started today....

Stagnant Water is of alcohol and yeast production, many of us have high amounts of background fermentation because of the high amounts of biofilms we have!!!

Muscle literally moves with and because of fascia, lack of exercise plus dehydration cause the tissues to stick and then soon as you attempt to move... POP! THE ONLY WAY TO STAY CLEAN AND LUBED UP IS

PERPETUAL MOTION!

The feet, ankles, lower spine fascia are loaded with mechanoreceptors. Mechanoreceptors are the fastest working Neurons/Nerves in the human body. They carry the most urgent messages, pain, fast movement etc... The instincts to dodge a punch or car etc... when you need each second to count... Those are mechanoreception, the fascia is loaded with them in fact **only the fascia has more nerve than the skin**!

Thoracolumbar Fascia - The TLF is a critical part of a myofascial girdle that surrounds the lower portion of the torso, playing an important role in posture, load transfer and respiration. [1] The fascial system is a "fibrous collagenous tissue which is part of a body-wide tensional force transmission system".Carla Stecco, says "the thoracolumbar fascia is like a large receptor that can sense tension coming from the arms, legs, spine, and abdominal cavity."

Tension here is registered as pain so no pain no gain does have some traction here... Many people experiencing lower back pain have thick, sticky, dehydrated fascia! This is the purpose of interoception, internal information processing. We just have to stop ignoring our body's many cries for help!

The Fascia form the fastest means of communication for all tissue via the nerves and interstitium, this basically the biomolecules that are in the various feathers. Think of these feathers like wine cases, any movement shakes all the wines up, even those movements are communications. Remember we discuss fiber optics and copper wires, the fascia is a combination of the two. It bridges the gaps between all other systems and is yet another reason why...

God is Music!

MORE FACTS…

Mesentery - a 'New' organ

J Calvin Coffey 1 2, Dara Walsh 1 2, Kevin G Byrnes 1 2, Werner Hohenberger 3, Richard J Heald 4 5
Affiliations expand

· PMID: 32539112 DOI: 10.1042/ETLS20200006

Abstract

The mesentery is the organ in which all abdominal digestive organs develop, and which maintains these in systemic continuity in adulthood. Interest in the mesentery was rekindled by advancements of Heald and Hohenberger in colorectal surgery. Conventional descriptions hold there are multiple mesenteries centrally connected to the posterior midline. Recent advances first demonstrated that, distal to the duodenojejunal flexure, the mesentery is a continuous collection of tissues. This observation explained how the small and large intestines are centrally connected, and the anatomy of the associated peritoneal landscape. In turn it prompted recategorisation of the mesentery as an organ. Subsequent work demonstrated the mesentery remains continuous throughout development, and that abdominal digestive organs (i.e. liver, spleen, intestine and pancreas) develop either on, or in it. This relationship is retained into adulthood when abdominal digestive organs are directly connected to the mesentery (i.e. they are 'mesenteric' in embryological origin and anatomical position). Recognition of mesenteric continuity identified the mesenteric model of abdominal anatomy according to which all abdominal abdomino-pelvic organs are organised into either a mesenteric or a non-mesenteric domain. This model explains the positional anatomy of all abdominal digestive organs, and associated vasculature. Moreover, it explains the peritoneal landscape and enables differentiation of peritoneum from the mesentery. Increased scientific focus on the mesentery has identified multiple vital or specialised functions. These vary across time and in anatomical location. The following review demonstrates how recent advances related to the mesentery are re-orientating the study of human biology in general and, by extension, clinical practice.

Bitter taste receptor (TAS2R) 46 in human skeletal muscle: expression and activity

Maria Talmon, 1 Erika Massara, 1 Martina Quaregna, 1 Marta De Battisti, 1 Francesca Boccafoschi, 1 Giulia Lecchi, 1 Federico Puppo, 1 Michele A. Bettega Cajandab, 1 Stefano Salamone, 2 Enrica Bovio, 1 Renzo Boldorini, 1 Beatrice Riva, 2 Federica Pollastro, 2 and Luigia G. Fresu 1 ,*

Author information Article notes Copyright and License information PMC Disclaimer

Associated Data

Supplementary Materials
Data Availability Statement

Go to:

Abstract

Bitter taste receptors are involved not only in taste perception but in various physiological functions as their anatomical location is not restricted to the gustatory system. We previously demonstrated expression and activity of the subtype hTAS2R46 in human airway smooth muscle and broncho-epithelial cells, and here we show its expression and functionality in human skeletal muscle cells. Three different cellular models were used: micro-dissected human skeletal tissues, human myoblasts/ myotubes and human skeletal muscle cells differentiated from urine stem cells of healthy donors. We used qPCR, immunohistochemistry and immunofluorescence analysis to evaluate gene and protein hTAS2R46 expression. In order to explore receptor activity, cells were incubated with the specific bitter ligands absinthin and 3ß-hydroxydihydrocostunolide, and calcium oscillation and relaxation were evaluated by calcium imaging and collagen assay, respectively, after a cholinergic stimulus. We show, for the first time, experimentally the presence and functionality of a type 2 bitter receptor in human skeletal muscle cells. Given the tendentially protective role of the bitter receptors starting from the oral cavity and following also in the other ectopic sites, and given its expression already at the myoblast level, we hypothesize that the bitter receptor can play an important role in the development, maintenance and in the protection of muscle tissue functions.

Keywords: bitter taste receptor, skeletal muscle, urine stem cells, urine stem cell-derived skeletal muscle cells, absinthin, calcium imaging

Go to:

1 Introduction

Bitterness perception is an innate aversive sense and is therefore a defence mechanism against potentially toxic substances. Indeed, bitter taste receptors (TAS2R) are mainly expressed in the oral cavity to protect us from ingesting anything that is potentially poisonous (Chandrashekar et al., 2000; Chaudhari and Roper, 2010). However, several in vitro and in vivo studies have investigated the extra chemoreceptive roles of TAS2Rs in extra-oral tissues, as well as their possible clinical implications (Jeruzal-Świątecka et al., 2020; Tuzim and Korolczuk, 2021; An and Liggett, 2018; Jaggupilli et al., 2017; Carey and Lee, 2019). The expression of hTAS2Rs is documented ectopically in a number of tissues, including the gut and stomach, the genitourinary system, the brain, the heart, the bone, white blood cells and the respiratory airways (Grassin-Delyle et al., 2013; Liszt et al., 2017; Rozengurt, 2006; Bloxham et al., 2020; Chen et al., 2017; Cheng et al., 2021; Welcome, 2020; Malki et al., 2015; Talmon et al., 2022a), suggesting a role beyond mere taste perception (Lu et al., 2017). For example, activation of bitter receptors in lung leads to the facilitation of foreign body removal, by inducing an increase in mucus secretion and cilia beating (Talmon et al., 2020; Sharma et al., 2022), while in the contracted airways smooth muscle cells they induce an important bronchodilation (Talmon et al., 2019; Deshpande et al., 2010). In addition to the lung, the expression and function of the hTAS2 receptor in smooth muscle has also been described in other organs, also demonstrating its potential as a pharmacological target (Manson et al., 2014; Zheng et al.,

2017; Zhai et al., 2016; Sakai et al., 2016). TAS2R represents the second largest group (25 members) of chemosensory G-protein coupled receptors (GPCRs): in taste buds, the downstream signalling involves the dissociation of a-gustducin that then triggers PLCβ2 activation to cleave the phosphatidylinositol 4,5-bisphosphate (PIP2) into inositol 1,4,5-tri- phosphate (IP3) and diacylglycerol (DAG), followed by an increase in cytosolic calcium that leads to taste recognition in the brain (Ueda et al., 2003). Conversely, in ectopic sites the cytosolic calcium signalling pathway is strictly dependent not only on the tissue but also on the bitter agonist and the receptor under study (Talmon et al., 2022b; Lu et al., 2017; Wooding et al., 2021).

In previous work (Talmon et al., 2019; Talmon et al., 2020), while performing immunohistochemistry of tongue and lung sections, we serendipitously found that TAS2R46 was also located in the striae of skeletal muscle. Capitalizing on this evidence, we demonstrate for the first time both gene and protein expression of bitter taste receptor TAS2R46 in human skeletal muscle cells. Moreover, we show that its activation counteracts the increase in cytosolic calcium and consequent induced contraction of acetylcholine, leading us to hypothesize that this receptor may also have a protective role in skeletal muscle.

Go to:

2 Materials and methods

2.1 Absinthin isolation

A voucher specimen of the Pancalieri chemotype of Arthemisia absinthium is kept in Novara laboratories. 1,300 g of leaves and flowers, powdered, were extracted with acetone (3 × 7.5 L) in a vertical percolator at room temperature, affording 97 g (7.5%) of a dark green syrup. The acetonic extract was dissolved into the minimal amount of acetone at 45 C and then 97 g silica gel was added (ratio extract/silica 1:1), finally the suspension was evaporated. Then absinthin was isolated according to Beauhaire et al. (1980), whose structure elucidation and purity were confirmed from 1H NMR (Supplementary Figure S1).

2.2 Immunohistochemistry analysis

The immunohistochemistry analysis was performed on μm-thick sections of FFPE with DAKO Autostainer (Dako) platform. After diagnostic procedures, remaining sections of tongue and locomotor skeletal muscle biopsies were baked for 30 min at 60°C, deparaffinised with xylene and rehydrated using EtOH washes of decreasing concentrations. For epitope retrieval, slides were treated in preheated citrate buffer and microwaved for 12 min at 650 W. The endogenous peroxidase activity was blocked by incubation in 3% H2O2 for 5 min. The incubation with primary antibody was performed for 1 h at RT, using polyclonal rabbit anti-human hTAS2R46 (dilution 1:1,500, OSR00173W, ThermoFisher). Subsequently, the reaction was revealed with Envision Dual Rabbit/Mouse detection system, using 3'3-diaminobenzidine tetrahydrochloride (DAB) as chromogen. The slides were counterstained with hematoxylin. When investigating the expression on the locomotor system, we used digastric, scalene and sternocleidomastoid muscle sections.

2.3 Cell culture

2.3.1 Primary human myoblasts and myotubes Primary myoblasts were obtained from 1 mm3 fragments of muscle biopsies, as previously reported (Garibaldi et al., 2016). Collection of biopsies was carried out in accordance with the policies of Sapienza University, and with The Code of Ethics of the World Medical Association (Declaration of Helsinki). An informed written consent was obtained from the volunteers. Each fragment was placed in a 60 mm dish in phosphate-buffered saline (PBS), muscle bundles were then separated longitudinally and subsequently chopped into smaller pieces. The small fragments were trypsinized for 40 'at 37°C on a magnetic stirrer and the reaction neutralized by serum. Samples were then centrifuged and the pellet, resuspended in PBS, was then plated in DMEM (Invitrogen) supplemented with 20% FBS (Gibco). Eight to 10 days after, the first myoblasts were visible. The clones, visible to the naked eye, were then isolated using 5 mm cloning rings. Myoblasts were maintained in DMEM supplemented with 10% heat-inactivated FCS (Gibco, Italy), l-glutamine 50 mg/mL (Sigma-Aldrich, Italy), penicillin 10 U/mL, streptomycin 100 mg/mL (Sigma-Aldrich, Italy), and sodium pyruvate 1 mM at 37°C, under a 5% CO_2 humidified atmosphere for 6–7 days with a medium change every 24–36 h. In order to establish the myoblast cultures, we performed an immunocytochemistry assay with a desmin specific antibody (Sc-58745, Santa Cruz). For differentiation into myotubes, myoblasts were transferred for 24 h into differentiation medium consisting of DMEM with 5% horse serum and 1% penicillin-streptomycin and sodium pyruvate 1 mM and then further maintained in the same medium for a further 24 h upon plating onto glass coverslips at a concentration of 15×10^4 per mL (24 mm diameter coverslips in 6 well plates) and maintained in DMEM/5% FCS supplemented with 10% heat-inactivated FBS (Gibco, Italy), l-glutamine 50 mg/mL (Sigma-Aldrich, Italy), penicillin 10 U/mL, streptomycin 100 mg/mL (Sigma-Aldrich, Italy), and sodium pyruvate 1 mM at 37°C, under a 5% CO_2 humidified atmosphere. Experiments were performed at P2. Additionally, human primary skeletal muscle cells (SkMCs) were obtained from ATCC (catalog PCS-950-010). SkMCs were maintained in Mesenchymal Stem Cell Basal Medium (ATCC, catalog PCS-500-030) supplemented with Primary Skeletal Muscle Growth Kit (ATCC, catalog PCS-950-040). For differentiation into myotubes, cells were cultured 96 h with

Skeletal Muscle Differentiation Tool (PCS-950-050).

2.3.2 Urine-derived stem cells (USC) and differentiation to skeletal muscle cells (SkMCs) Collection of human urine from healthy volunteers was approved by the local Ethics Committee (Comitato Etico Interaziendale Maggiore della Carità, Novara; authorization CE 190/20), and the work was carried out in accordance with The Code of Ethics of the World Medical Association (Declaration of Helsinki) and an informed written consent was obtained from the volunteers. USCs were isolated from 13 urine samples (30–300 ml) collected from 5 healthy individuals (age from 23 to 35 years old). The samples were preserved with 10% primary medium (DMEM/F12, 10% FBS, 1% penicillin-streptomycin, 2.5 µg/ml amphotericin B - ThermoFisher-, renal epithelial growth medium SingleQuot supplement–LGC Standard) for 24 h at 4°C before the isolation. USCs were isolated and differentiated as previously described (Talmon et al., 2022a). Briefly, urine samples were centrifuged (10 'at 400 g) and the pellet washed twice in washing buffer. The obtained cells were plated in a 0.1% gelatin coated-24-well plate in 500 µl of primary medium. 24, 48 and 72 h later 500 µl of primary medium were added. Then, 1.5 ml of medium were removed and 500 µl of proliferation medium were added. The half of the medium was daily changed. For differentiation into skeletal muscle cells (SkMCs), sub-confluent USCs (P2-P4) were transduced with a second-generation lentiviral vector carrying an inducible MyoD insert (LV-TRE-VP64 human MyoD-T2A-dsRedExpress2), that was a gift from Charles Gersbach (Addgene plasmid # 60629; http://n2t.net/addgene:60629; RRID:Addgene_60629) (Kabadi et al., 2015), plated on mouse collagen I-coated plates in differentiation medium and cultured for 28 days. Medium was changed daily. 72 h before experiments medium was changed with a differentiation medium without horse serum and containing 5% FBS (Gibco).

2.4 RNA isolation and qPCR

Total RNA was isolated by Trizol (ThermoFisher) from USCs, USC-SkMCs, primary myoblasts and myotubes, skeletal muscle biopsies from tongue and locomotor system. The amount and purity of total RNA were quantified at the spectrophotometer (Nanodrop, Thermo Fisher) by measuring the optical density at 260 and 280 nm. 1μg of total RNA was reverse-transcribed using a high-capacity SensiFAST™ cDNA Synthesis Kit (Bioline) according to the manufacturer's instructions. For quantitative polymerase chain reaction (qPCR) gene specific primers (Supplementary Table S1) and TaqMan Expression Assay (hTAS2R46; Applied Biosystems) were used. TAS2Rs screening was performed with iTaq Universal SYBR Green Supermix (Biorad). For TaqMan assay, TaqMan Universal PCR MasterMix (2×) (without AmpErase UNG; Applied Biosystem) was used with a 7000 ABI Prism system (Applied Biosystems) was used. Glyceraldehyde-3-phosphate dehydrogenase (GAPDH) and β-glucuronidase (GUSβ) were the endogenous controls; nicotinic acetylcholine receptor subunits (nACHRa4 and nACHRa9) were used as positive control, cytokeratin 10 (CK10) as negative control.

2.5 Immunofluorescence

2×10^5 cells were plated on 12 mm Ø glass dish, fixed in PAF 4% for 10' and then incubated with the blocking buffer (3% BSA, 0.1% Triton X-100 in PBS) for 1 h at room temperature (RT). Cells were then incubated with polyclonal rabbit anti-human hTAS2R46 (OSR00173W, Thermo Fisher) primary antibody for 2 h at RT and then incubated for 45 'at RT in the dark with the secondary antibody goat anti-rabbit AlexaFluor 488 (Thermo Fisher). For nuclei and cytoskeleton staining DAPI and TRITC-phalloidin (Sigma-Aldrich) were added to the secondary antibody solution.

2.6 Lentiviral vectors production for hTAS2R46 shRNA

hTAS2R46 expression in USCs-SkMCs was silenced by lentiviral infection. Two lentiviral constructs targeting hTAS2R46 (TCRN0000014110 and TCRN0000014112) were obtained from TRCHs1.0 library (Dharmacon). Third-generation LVs were produced co-transfecting HEK293T packaging cells with plasmids pMDLg/pRRE, pMD2. VSVG, pRSV-Rev and transfer construct using the Lipofectamine 2000 (Invitrogen), as described previously (Talmon et al., 2019). USC-SkMCs were then transduced with the LV-shRNAs together and the silencing was assessed by qPCR.

2.7 Membrane potential analysis

For membrane potential analysis, SkMCs were loaded for 30 min at RT in the dark with a voltage-sensitive dye using the FluoVolt Membrane Potential Kit (Thermo Fisher), following manufacturer instructions, and the fluorescence were evaluated at the cyotofluorimeter (Attune NxT–Thermo Fisher). 20.000 were acquired to set basal conditions and then stimulated with absinthin (10 µM) and acetylcholine (100 µM) alone or combined. Data were expressed and analysed as delta of mean fluorescence intensity (MFI) before and after the stimulus.

2.8 Calcium imaging analysis

USCs and USC-SkMCs were plated on a pre-coated glass coverslip with 0.1% gelatin and collagen type I, respectively. For evaluation of Ca2+ fluctuations, cells were loaded with 5 µM Fura-2 a.m. (ThermoFisher) in the presence of 0.02% Pluronic-127 and 10 µM sulfinpyrazone in Krebs–Ringer buffer (KRB; 135 mM NaCl, 5 mM KCl, 0.4 mM KH2PO4, 1 mM MgSO4, 5.5 mM glucose, 20 mM HEPES, pH 7.4) containing 2 mM CaCl2 (30 min, RT). Then, cells were washed and incubated with KRB for 30 min to allow the de-esterification of Fura-2 a.m. For measurements of mitochondrial Ca2+, cells were loaded with Rhod-2a.m. (ThermoFisher) in the presence of 0.2% Pluronic-127 in KRB containing 2 mM CaCl2 (30 min, RT) and then incubated with KRB for 1 h to allow the de-esterification. The basal calcium was monitored for about 50 s and then cells were challenged with the following stimuli alone ore combined: acetylcholine (Ach, 100 µM; Sigma-Aldrich), absinthin (Abs 1, 10, 100 µM, 1 mM), cynaropicrin (10, 10 µM, 1 mM), strychnine (10, 10 µM, 1 mM), 3β-hydroxydihydrocostunolide (3-HDC, 1, 10, 100 µM, Sigma-Aldrich), H-89 dihydrochloride PKA inhibitor (10 µm, Sigma-Aldrich), ESI-09 (a pan-EPAC inhibitor, 10 µm, Sigma-Aldrich), and KB-R7943 carbamimidothioic-acid (KB, 10 µm, Sigma-Aldrich). During the experiments, coverslips were mounted into an acquisition chamber and placed on the stage of a Leica DMI6000 epifluorescent microscope equipped with S Fluor ×40/1.3 objective. Fura-2 a.m. was excited by alternating 340 nm and 380 nm using a Polychrome IV monochromator (Till Photonics, Germany), and the probe emission light was filtered through a 520/20 bandpass filter and collected by a cooled CCD camera (Hamamatsu, Japan). Rhod-2a.m. was excited at 552 nm and the fluorescence emission was recorded at 580 nm. The fluorescence signals were acquired and processed using MetaFluor software (Molecular Devices, United States). To quantify the differences in the amplitudes of Ca2+ transients, the Fura-2a.m. and Rhod-2a.m. fluorescences were expressed relative to the fluorescence intensity at the stimulation time ($\Delta F/F0$).

2.9 Contraction assay

USC-SkMCs and primary SkMCs (400.000 cells/mL) were embedded in collagen gel (mouse tail, final concentration of 8 mg/mL) with or without acetylcholine (100 µM), absinthin (10 µM), PKA inhibitor (H89, 10 µM) and EPAC inhibitor (ESI-09, 10 µM) and seeded in triplicate for each condition in 24-well plates. After solidification, the gels were incubated in DMEM with 5% FBS and stimuli. Cells were left to grow, and area of collagen disk was measured from 1 h to 72 h after cells reached the confluence.

2.10 Statistical analysis

Statistical analyses were performed using GraphPad Prism 5 (California, United States). Data are presented mean ±SEM of 'n'independent experiments performed in triplicate. Data were analysed by one-way ANOVA. To adjust for multiple testing and to assess differences between control group and each of the treatment we have applied the Dunn's test. A value of $p < 0.05$ was considered statistically significant.

Go to:

3 Results

3.1 Expression of hTAS2R46 in human skeletal tissue

The expression of the 25 human bitter taste receptor subtypes was evaluated on skeletal muscle biopsies from the locomotor system and oral cavity. As shown by qPCR analysis (Figure 1A; Supplementary Table S1) several isoforms of the bitter taste receptor are expressed in skeletal muscle, among which TAS2R46 appears to be the most representative (Figure 1A). Immunohistochemistry analysis confirmed and highlighted that the TAS2R46 protein is well expressed all along the striated skeletal muscle fibres of both locomotor system (Figure 1B) and tongue (Figure 1C). The stain with the secondary antibody only (Figure 1E) demonstrates the specificity of the primary antibody and therefore the reliability of the receptor expression.

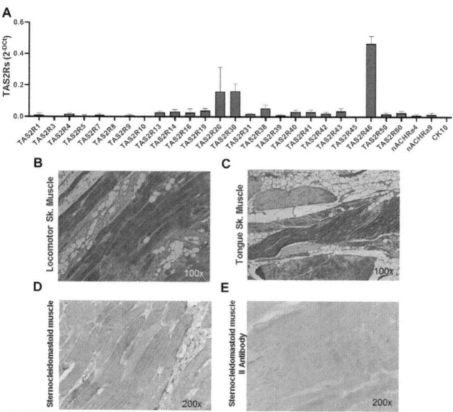

FIGURE 1

Expression of hTAS2Rs in human skeletal muscle biopsies. (A) qPCR analysis of hTAS2R subtypes expression in human biopsies (n = 4) of skeletal muscles (oral cavity and locomotor system). Nicotinic acetylcholine receptor subunits (nACHRa4 and nACHRa9) were used as positive control, cytokeratin 10 (CK10) as negative control. Data are expressed as 2-DCt and are means ±SEM. (B, C) Immunohistochemistry analysis of TAS2R46 expression on sections of locomotor system (B) and tongue (C) skeletal muscle. Magnification ×100. Positive (stained with both primary and secondary antibody, (D) and negative (stained with secondary antibody only, (E) control of immunohistochemistry analysis of section of sternoclaidomastoid skeletal muscle.

3.2 Expression of hTAS2R46 in human myoblast/myotube

Both myoblasts from skeletal muscle biopsies and primary SkMC line were subcultured and differentiated into mature myotubes. hTAS2R46 expression level was evaluated in both cell types. As observed by immunofluorescence assay (**Figure**

2; Supplementary Figure S2) the receptor was detected in both myoblasts (Figures 2A, C) and myotubes (Figures 2B, D), with the difference that in myoblasts it was mainly localized in the perinuclear area while in the myotubes it was expressed predominantly on the cell surface. Moreover, levels of mRNA increased considerably during the differentiation process (Figure 2E; Supplementary Figure S2).

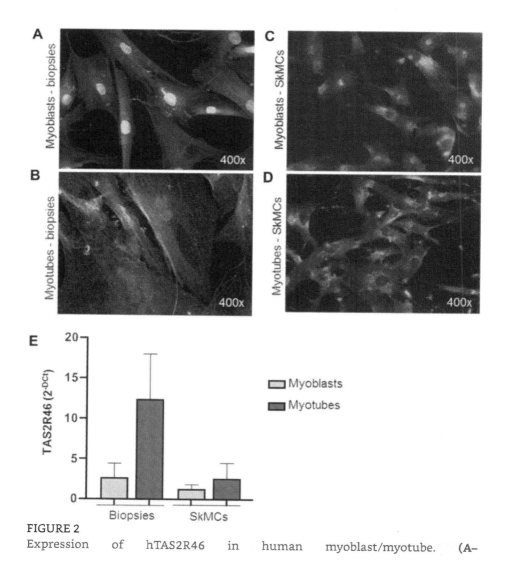

FIGURE 2

Expression of hTAS2R46 in human myoblast/myotube. **(A–**

D) Immunofluorescence analysis of TAS2R46 expression in myoblasts **(A)** and myotubes **(B)** isolated from biopsies and primary SkMCs before **(C)** and after **(D)** last step of differentiation. Green: TAS2R46; Blue: Nuclei; Red. Magnification ×400. **(E)** Real time analysis of TAS2R46 expression on myoblasts and myotubes from biopsies and a primary cell line of SkMCs. Data are expressed as 2-DCt and are means ±SEM of at least three independent experiments.

3.3 Expression of hTAS2R46 in USCs and USC-derived skeletal muscle cells

Functional characterization of primary myoblasts/myotubes is hampered by both technical and ethical issues. Therefore, we took advantage of USC-derived skeletal muscle cells (USC-SkMCs), a well characterized skeletal muscle cellular model established in our laboratory (**Talmon et al., 2022b**). As shown in **Figure 3**, expression of hTAS2R46 was demonstrated by immunofluorescence analysis also in this system (**Figures 3A, B**). We evaluated gene expression in both USC and USC-SkMCs and it is noteworthy the significant increase of hTAS2R46 expression after differentiation (**Figure 3C; Supplementary Figure S2**).

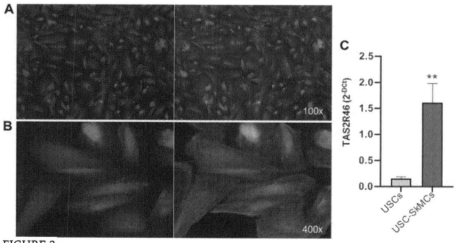

FIGURE 3
Expression of hTAS2R46 in USC-SkMCs. **(A–B)** Immunofluorescence analysis of TAS2R46 expression USC-SkMCs. Green: TAS2R46; Blue: Nuclei; Red: Phalloidin. Magnification ×100 and 400x. **(C)** Real-time PCR analysis of TAS2R46 gene transcript expression in USCs and USC-SkMCs. Data are expressed as 2-DCt and are means ±SEM of five independent experiments. $**p < 0.01$ vs. USCs.

3.4 hTAS2R46 was functional in skeletal muscle cells

To evaluate whether hTAS2R46 was functional in skeletal muscle, we treated cells with absinthin, its most selective and potent agonist (**Talmon et al., 2019**), and two non-specific bitter tastants, strychnine and cynaropicrin. Absinthin was unable to induce a measurable increase of cytosolic calcium by itself at the lowest concentration tested (10 μM), although at higher concentrations a dose-dependent cytosolic calcium release could be observed (**Supplementary Figure S3**). The same trend and rank order of potency were observed treating cells with strychnine, while cynaropicrin gave a stronger effect reaching the maximum calcium peak at 100 μM (**Supplementary Figure S3**).

3.5 Absinthin modulates acetylcholine-induced response skeletal muscle cells

We then evaluated the effect of the absinthin on the membrane potential and on calcium variations induced by one of the major pro-contractile neurotransmitters, acetylcholine (100 μM). As shown in **Figure 4**, acetylcholine induced a rapid membrane potential transient that was reverted by co-stimulation with absinthin. Moreover, Fura-2a.m. analysis demonstrated that acetylcholine induced a rapid increase in cytosolic calcium (**Figures 5A, B**) which was counteracted by absinthin, already at the lowest concentration tested (1–100 μM, **Figure 5A**). The effect of absinthin on acetylcholine-induced Ca^{2+}-rises was strictly dependent on hTAS2R46 activation since it was reversed by 3HDC, a specific antagonist of this receptor (**Brockhoff et al., 2011**) (**Figure 5B**), and was completely abolished in USC-SkMCs silenced for TAS2R46 expression (**Figure 5C; Supplementary Figure S4**).

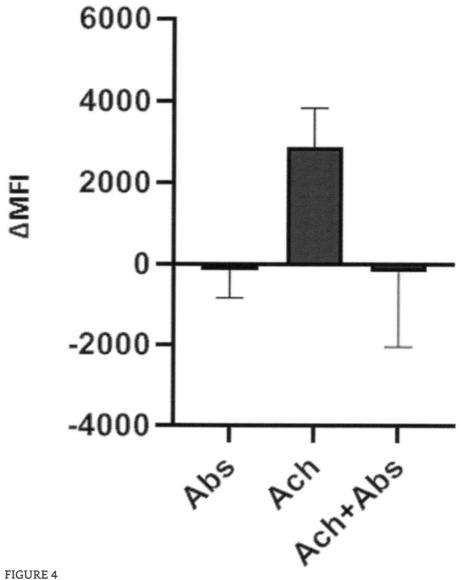

FIGURE 4
Membrane potential modulation by absinthin and acetylcholine. Human primary myotubes were charged with FluoVolt membrane dye and the variations in the fluorescence intensity were evaluated at the cytofluorimeter. Data are illustrated in histograms representing the mean ±SEM of the mean fluorescence intensity variations (ΔMFI) before and after cells stimulation with acetylcholine (100 μM) and absinthin (10 μM) alone or combined (n = 5).

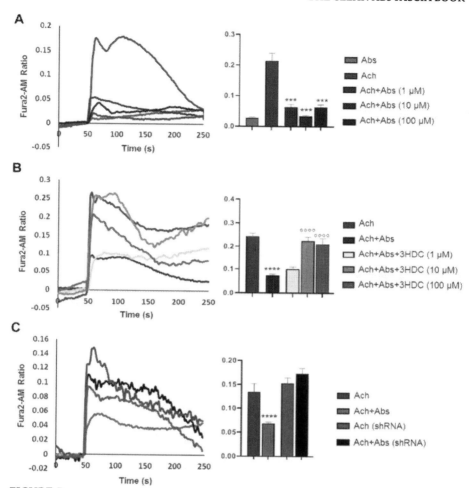

FIGURE 5

Absinthin reduces acetylcholine-induced Ca2+ transients in a TAS2R46-dependent manner. Data are illustrated in representative traces as well as in histogram expressing the mean ±SEM of maximum peak of cytosolic Ca2+ release of at least 32 cells in three independent experiments. (A) Fura-2a.m.–loaded USC-SkMCs were stimulated with acetylcholine (Ach) 100 µm and absinthin (Abs) 10 µm alone or combined. ****$p < 0.001$ vs. Ach. (B) USC-SkMCs were stimulated with acetylcholine (Ach) 100 µm, absinthin (Abs) 10 µm and increasing concentrations of receptor antagonist 3HDC (1, 10, 100 µm). ****$p < 0.0001$ vs. Ach; **** $p < 0.0001$ vs. Ach + Abs. (C) Fura-2a.m.-loaded USC-SkMCs silenced for hTAS2R46 expression (referred as shRNA) were stimulated with acetylcholine (Ach) 100 µm, absinthin (Abs) 10 µm alone ore combined.

3.6 Absinthin modulated acetylcholine-calcium rise in a

cAMP-dependent manner

We previously demonstrated that in airway smooth muscle cells absinthin counteracts histamine-induced calcium rise, in a similar manner to what observed with acetylcholine in skeletal muscle, stimulating mitochondrial Ca_{2+}-uptake in a cAMP/EPAC dependent way (**Talmon et al., 2019**). To test whether this mechanism was present also in skeletal muscle, we recorded the cytosolic calcium oscillation in USC-SkMCs stimulated with acetylcholine alone or combined with absinthin, in the presence of a PKA inhibitor (H-89, 10 μM) or a specific EPAC inhibitor (ESI-09, 10 μM). As shown in **Figure 6**, both the co-stimulation with H-89 and ESI-09 abolished the ability of absinthin to reduce acetylcholine-induced calcium increases (**Figure 6**), demonstrating therefore a direct involvement of the cAMP/EPAC cascade in the downstream signalling of hTAS2R46. Since Epac1 is localized on the mitochondrial inner membrane and matrix and can control the activity of the mitochondrial calcium uniporter (MCU) (**Faza et al., 2017; Wang et al., 2016**), we analysed the calcium movements in USC-SkMCs co-stimulated with acetylcholine, absinthin and the MCU inhibitor KB-R7943 (carbamimidothioic acid, KB, 10 μM). Again, KB-R7043 treatment resulted in a complete inhibition of the effect of absinthin (**Figure 6**, yellow line and bar).

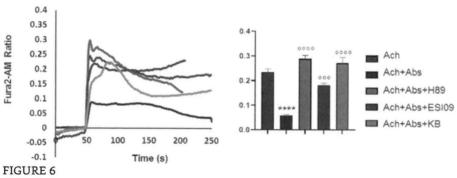

FIGURE 6

Absinthin reduces acetylcholine-induced Ca_{2+} transients via cAMP in USC-SkMCs. Data are illustrated in representative traces as well as in histogram expressing the mean ±SEM of maximum peak of cytosolic Ca2+ release of at least 54 cells in three independent experiments. Fura-2a.m.–loaded USC-SkMCs were stimulated with acetylcholine (Ach) 100 μm, absinthin (Abs) 1 μM in presence of the PKA inhibitor H-89 (10 μM), or a pan-EPAC inhibitor (ESI-09, 10 μm) or MCU inhibitor KB-R7943 (10 μm). ****$p < 0.0001$ vs. Ach; *** $p < 0.001$**** $p < 0.0001$ vs. Ach + Abs.

3.7 Absinthin induced mitochondrial calcium uptake

The above data would suggest that absinthin signals via cAMP/EPAC to the mitochondrial MCU to increase the uptake of Ca2+. If this were the case, it could be expected that the reduction in cytosolic calcium would be paralleled by a simultaneous increase in calcium within the mitochondria. We then evaluated mitochondrial calcium levels by Rhod2-AM analysis. As expected, acetylcholine determined a mild increase in mitochondrial calcium that was significantly augmented by the co-stimulation with absinthin (**Figure 7**, red and blue lines and bars). The effect was completely reverted by 3HDC, confirming that the effect is strictly dependent on hTAS2R46 (**Figure 7**; light blue line and bar), and by the MCU inhibitor (**Figure 7**; yellow line and bar). Moreover, the effect of absinthin was counteracted by the incubation with H-89 and ESI-09, confirming the involvement of cAMP in the downstream cascade and perfectly aligning the effects obtained on cytosolic Ca2+ to those on mitochondrial Ca2+.

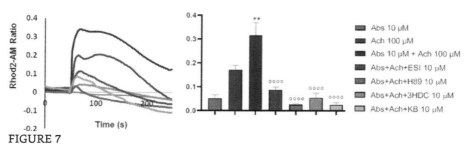

FIGURE 7

Absinthin increased mithocondrial Ca2+ entry. Data are illustrated in representative traces as well as in histogram expressing the mean ±SEM of maximum peak of cytosolic Ca2+ release of at least 43 cells in three independent experiments. Rhod-2a.m.–loaded USC-SkMCs were stimulated with acetylcholine (Ach) 100 μm, absinthin (Abs) 1 μM in presence of the antagonist 3HDC (10 μm), or the PKA inhibitor H-89 (10 μM), or the pan-EPAC inhibitor (ESI-09, 10 μm) or MCU inhibitor KB-R7943 (10 μm). **$p < 0.01$ vs. Ach; **** $p < 0.0001$ vs. Ach + Abs.

3.8 Bitter agonist induces relaxation effect on USC-SkMCs

The above results, alongside providing further evidence for a novel signalling pathway that decreases Ca_{2+}-signalling via increasing mitochondrial uptake, also suggest that hTAS2R46 activation might influence acetylcholine-induced contraction. We therefore tested this hypothesis in the collagen contraction assay. Skeletal muscle cells are spontaneously endowed of contraction and therefore even in absence of stimuli (**Figure 8, no stimuli**) it possible to measure a slight reduction of the collagen disc diameter. Interestingly, absinthin, alone, did not stimulate the contraction of USC-SkMCs, as demonstrated by a contraction kinetics superimposable to that of unstimulated cells (**Figure 8A**). As expected, acetylcholine, amplified and fastened the contraction process as early as 3 h after the addition of the neurotransmitter (**Figure 8A**), significantly shrinking the collagen disk, in comparison to control cells (**Figure 8C**). The co-stimulation with absinthin and acetylcholine slowed down the kinetic of the acetylcholine-induced contraction, and after 6 h the collagen area was still significantly larger than that of the acetylcholine-stimulated cells (**Figures 8A, B**). To further understand the machinery involved in the transduction signal, we performed the collagen contraction assay on primary SkMCs in the presence of both EPAC and PKA inhibitors: both compounds confirmed the ability of absinthin to contrast acetylcholine-induced contraction and strengthens the hypothesis that TAS2R46 mediates muscle dilation via cAMP (**Figures 8D, E**). Indeed, the EPAC inhibitor ESI-09 partially reverted absinthin effect between 3 and 4 h after contraction induction (**Figure 8E**).

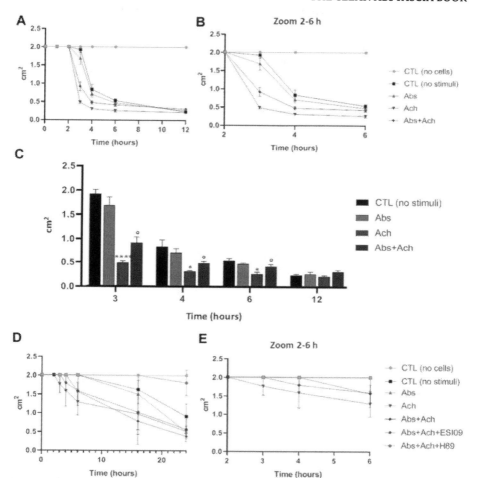

FIGURE 8

Absinthin counteracted acetylcholine-induced USC-SkMCs contraction. Cells were plated on collagen disc and treated with absinthin 10 μM, acetylcholine 100 μM. **(A)** The collagen area was measured at the indicated time point; **(B)** zoom of the time between the second and the fourth hours. **(C)** Histograms represent the mean ±SEM of collagen area (cm2) at several time points (n = 4) ****$p < 0.0001$; *$p < 0.05$ vs CTL (no stimuli); ° $p < 0.05$ vs Ach. **(D)** SkMCs were stimulated with absinthin 10 μM and acetylcholine 100 μM, also in presence of the PKA inhibitor (H89, 10 μM) and EPAC inhibitor (ESI-09); in **(E)** zoom of the time between the second and the fourth hours.

Go to:

4 Discussion

In the present report, using qPCR, immunohistochemistry, and immunofluorescence, we experimentally demonstrate the expression of several subtype of bitter taste receptor in human skeletal muscle cells, of which the subtype TAS2R46 showed the highest level of expression. Previously, the presence of TAS2R46 could have been hypothesized from microarrays performed on skeletal muscle (Gene Expression Omnibus), but no formal proof of its presence had been undertaken. Furthermore, we also show that TAS2R46 is functional, its activity is coupled to EPAC activation, and it antagonizes acetylcholine contraction. Because no TAS2R type had previously been demonstrated to be expressed on human skeletal muscle, we verified the expression and functionality of TAS2R46 by several different methods. While the definition of TAS2R46 as a key player in human muscle contraction is entirely novel, our results are corroborated by previous findings in rodents that suggested that bitter taste receptors might be present. Indeed, Zagorchev et al. (2019) showed that low concentrations of denatonium reduce *in vitro* the contraction of rat abdominal muscle preparations, and Kimura and Kato, (2020) the following year demonstrated the expression of different isoforms of TAS2R in murine skeletal muscle tissues and cell line, hypothesizing a role for these receptors related to metabolic functions. In human the expression of taste receptor family members has been reviewed in different non-gustatory system, both for TAS1R and TAS2R (Yamamoto and Ishimaru, 2013; Mennella et al., 2013) but so far only the former has been shown to be expressed and active in skeletal muscle. In skeletal muscle, expression of TAS1R appears to increase during differentiation, from myoblast to myocyte (Kokabu et al., 2015), and its function appears to be the sensing of nutrients, such as amino acids, and the regulation of the autophagy (Kokabu et al., 2017; Wauson et al., 2012), two critical processes for skeletal muscle function, thus suggesting that altered expression of this receptor may be involved in muscle pathologies such as sarcopenia, characterized by an incorrect autophagy (Kokabu et al., 2017). Our data show that TAS2R46 is also developmentally controlled and is expressed at higher levels in mature skeletal muscle cells. We next sought to determine the functionality of TAS2R46 by evaluating calcium activity and our results show its role in reducing contraction via a distinctive mechanism, by controlling ER/mitochondrial synapses at the MCU via a cAMP/EPAC pathway, in analogy to what previously reported in airway smooth muscle cells (Talmon et al., 2019).

As previously shown also in smooth muscle (Talmon et al., 2019), TAS2R46 activation does not disclose a direct effect alone but only in the presence of Ca_{2+}-mobilizing transmitters. Indeed, we can observe a significant decrease in cytosolic calcium and a concomitant increase in mitochondrial buffering. While the Ca_{2+}-handling capacity of the sarco (endo)plasmic reticulum outweighs that of mitochondria, this Ca_{2+}-shuttling is significant, as shown by the Ca_{2+}-traces and has repercussions on contraction. The importance of mitochondria in shaping Ca_{2+}-signals has been long known (Rizzuto et al., 2012) and it is also likely that this increased Ca_{2+} also alters mitochondrial bioenergetics, although we did not directly investigate it. In skeletal muscle, the importance of mitochondrial Ca_{2+} is less characterized than in other cell types but is important to note that mutations of the proteins involved in mitochondrial Ca_{2+}-transport have been very recently shown to lead to muscle dysfunction (Bulthuis, et al., 2022) providing evidence that this mechanism is highly relevant.

It would seem highly peculiar that during evolution such a sophisticated mechanism was conserved or found its place in skeletal muscle without a specific role, which we envisage being mediating fatigue or abnormal muscle contraction. Moreover, this physiological effect of absinthin in calcium modulation is so rapid that it could be interpreted as a protective response. The fact that TAS2R46 does not exclude that other bitter receptors may also be present, and their role and interplay will be of great interest to explore in the future. Indeed, we can speculate a synergy between TAS1R and TAS2R in skeletal muscle, as hypothesized by Carey et al. in cancer cells (Carey et al., 2022): on the one hand TAS1R may sensitise muscle towards nutrients, while on the other hand TAS2R may maintain calcium homeostasis avoiding cellular overwork. Therefore, our finding provides the perspective of this receptor as a target for antagonists to decrease muscle fatigue in disorders characterized by this, including dystrophies. The question arises, though, on which endogenous (bitter) compound would trigger the activation of these receptors.

Bitter Taste Receptors as Regulators of Abdominal Muscles Contraction

P. ZAGORCHEV,[1,4] G. V. PETKOV,[2] and H. S. GAGOV[3]
Author information Copyright and License information PMC Disclaimer

The publisher's final edited version of this article is available free at Physiol Res

Go to:

Summary

Bitter taste receptors (TAS2R) are expressed in many non-sensor tissues including skeletal muscles but their function remains unexplored. The aim of this study is to investigate the role of TAS2R in rat abdominal skeletal muscles contractions using denatonium, a TAS2R agonist. Low concentration of denatonium (0.01 mmol/l) caused a significant decrease of amplitudes of the electrical field stimulation (EFS)-induced contractions in abdominal skeletal muscles preparations *in vitro*. This inhibitory effect was significantly reduced when the preparations were pre-incubated with gentamicin (0.02 mmol/l) used as a non-specific inhibitor of IP_3 formation or with $BaCl_2$ (0.03 mmol/l) applied to block the inward-rectifier potassium current. All experiments were performed in the presence of pipecuronium in order to block the nerve stimulation of the contractions. The data obtained suggest that denatonium decreases the force of rat abdominal muscles contractions mainly *via* activation of TAS2R, phosphatidylinositol 4,5-biphosphate and its downstream signal metabolites.

Keywords: Skeletal muscle, Taste receptors, Electric field stimulation, PIP_2, IP_3, Relaxation

Go to:

Introduction

Sweet, umami and bitter taste receptors are widely expressed in non-taste sensory organs. Bitter taste receptors (TAS2R) are involved in the regulation of the physiological processes such as airway smooth muscle cell relaxation and bronchodilation, the secretion of the gastro-intestinal tract, artery relaxation, as well as in the modulation of nervous and immune systems (for review Dalesio *et al.* 2018). These influences are supposed to be related to TAS2R signal pathway which activates G-protein, phospholipase C (PLC), protein kinase C (PKC) and IP_3-induced Ca_{2+} release (IICR) in non-taste sensory tissues (Avau *et al.* 2015, Dalesio *et al.* 2018). As a result of this stimulation, cytoplasmic Ca_{2+} concentration increases and several protein targets of PKC change their activities. However, the effects of TAS2R activation in skeletal muscles remain unclear. The aim of this study is to investigate the effect of denatonium, an agonist of TAS2R, on electrical field stimulation (EFS)-induced abdominal skeletal muscles contractions and their dependence on phosphatidylinositol 4,5-bisphosphate (PIP2) and its break down. The role of inward-rectifier potassium (Kir) channels on TAS2R-induced effect was also studied.

Go to:

Materials and Methods

The experiments were approved by the Bulgarian Food Safety Agency and the Ethics Committee of the Medical University of Plovdiv, Bulgaria (approval nos. 87/9.01.2014 and 5/29.09.2016 respectively). Male Wistar rat *transversus abdominis muscles* strips were isometrically fixed as previously described (Zagorchev *et al.* 2016). During a period of 20 min the muscle activity was elicited by unipolar EFS used as a control and analysed (Zagorchev *et al.*, 2018). EFS were repeated, square-wave multipulses of supramaximal intensity, 0.5 ms in duration applied at frequency of 5 Hz and 50 Hz for 3 s followed by a 7 s pause. After this, denatonium 10^{-5} mol/l, gentamicin 2.10^{-5} mol/l, gentamicin 2.10^{-5} mol/l and denatonium 10^{-5} mol/l, $BaCl_2$ 3.10^{-5} mol/l or $BaCl_2$ 3.10^{-5} mol/l and denatonium 10^{-5} mol/l were added to the organ baths.

All experiments were conducted in the presence of 10-5 mol/l pipecuronium to block the nerve stimulation of the muscles (Youssef *et al.* 1993). For a statistical analysis, SPSS.15 (Chicago, IL, USA) was employed. All data are expressed as mean ± SEM after verifying the normality one-way analysis of variance (ANOVA), Bonferroni Multiple Comparison Test the Paired samples t-test. The number of tested muscle strips is indicated by *n*. Results were considered as statistically significant at $p<0.05$.

Go to:

Results

EFS-evoked (5 Hz) single contractions of rat *transversus abdominis muscles* preparations *in vitro* maintain stable but slightly declining amplitudes in the presence of pipecuronium, which was added to block the nerve stimulation of nicotinic acetylcholine receptor (nAChR, time control). Thus 1 min after drug application it was 5.2±0.5 mN, after 5 min – 4.7±0.5 mN and after 15 min – 4.1±0.4 mN (**Fig. 1 A,**

,B
B and

andC,
C, left column and **Fig. 2**, left panel, ж). The same event but less pronounced was observed in 50Hz EFS-evoked tetanic contractions (**Fig. 1D** and **Fig. 2**, right panel, ж). The addition of denatonium at a concentration of 10-5 mol/l induced a significant decrease (p<0.05, n=12) of the force of single contractions after 5 min to 1.7±0.6 mN and almost complete inhibition after 15 min (0.3±0.1 mN) along with a large decrease (p<0.05, n=12) of tetanic contractions after 15 min (2.3±0.5 mN) (**Fig. 2A**, ●). The inhibition of the contraction force was faster when 5.10-5 mol/l denatonium was used (data not shown). A low concentration of gentamicin (2.10-5 mol/l)

was applied into the bath to suppress selectively IP3 generation. This treatment also reduced the force of single and tetanic EFS-induced contractions but with a constant potency during the whole studied time interval (**Fig. 1**, **Fig. 2A**, ■). In the presence of simultaneously added 2.10-5 mol/l gentamicin and 10-5 mol/l denatonium (**Fig. 1**, **Fig. 2A**, ♦) a further decrease in the amplitudes of the contraction force was observed but the effect of denatonium was less pronounced as compared to the single contractions (p<0.05, n=12). Thus, the amplitudes of contractions after 5 min were 3.3±0.3 mN, after 10 min – 3.0±0.4 mN, after 15 min – 2.6±0.3 mN and at 20 min – 2.3±0.3 mN. For tetanic contractions, the denatonium suppression of the force of contraction in the presence of gentamicin was weaker: after 10 min it was 5.3±0.5 mN, after 15 min – 5.0±0.5 mN and after 20 min – 4.9±0.4 mN.

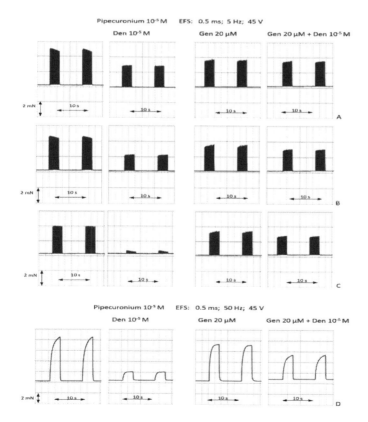

Fig. 1.

Direct EFS-evoked contractions of *m. transversus abdominis* preparations *in vitro* in the presence of 10-5 mol/l pipecuronium and after the addition of 10-5 mol/l denatonium (Den 10-5 M), of 2.10-5 mol/l gentamicin (Gen 20 µM) and of 10-5 mol/l denatonium and 2.10-5 mol/l gentamicin (Gen 20 µM + Den 10-5 M). **A)** after 1 min, **B)** after 5 min and **C)** after 15 min, all stimulated with EFS - 0.5 ms, 5Hz, 45V, **D)** 15 min after EFS with duration 0.5 ms, 50Hz, 45V.

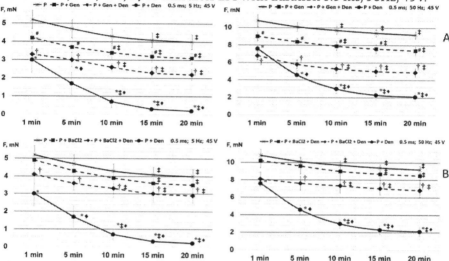

Fig. 2.

Time dependence of contraction force by direct EFS stimulation: 0.5ms, 5Hz, 45V – left and 0.5 ms, 50Hz, 45V – right. **A)** The curves represent the force in mN in the presence of 10-5 mol/l pipecuronium (P, ж) for a time control, of 10-5 mol/l pipecuronium and 2.10-5 mol/l gentamicin (P + Gen, ■), of 10-5 mol/l pipecuronium, 2.10-5 mol/l gentamicin and 10-5 mol/l denatonium (P + Gen + Den, ♦) and of 10-5 mol/l pipecuronium and denatonium (P + Den, ●), ‡ p< 0.05, n=12 vs effect on 1 min of the following measurements after 5, 10, 15 и 20 min, # p< 0.05 gentamicin *vs* time control, * p<0.05, n=12 denatonium *vs* time control, † p< 0.05 n=12 for denatonium *vs* gentamicin and ♦ p<0.05, n=12 for denatonium *vs* denatonium and gentamicin. **B)** The curves represent the force in mN in the presence of 10-5 mol/l pipecuronium (P, ж) for time control, of 10-5 mol/l pipecuronium and 3.10-5 mol/l BaCl2 (P + BaCl2, ■), of 10-5 mol/l pipecuronium, 3.10-5 mol/l BaCl2 and 10-5 mol/l denatonium (P + BaCl2 + Den, ♦) and of 10-5 mol/l pipecuronium and denatonium (P + Den, ●), ‡ p< 0.05, n=12 vs effect on 1 min of the following measurements after 5, 10, 15 and 20 min, # p< 0.05 BaCl2 *vs* time control, * p<0.05, n=12 denatonium *vs* time control, † p<0.05, n=12 for denatonium *vs* BaCl2 and ♦ p<0.05, n=12 for denatonium *vs* denatonium and BaCl2.

Next, we applied BaCl2 to inhibit Kir channels. In the presence of 0.03 mmol/l Ba^{2+} the maximal amplitudes of single contractions slightly declined after 5 min $BaCl_2$ application to 4.3±0.6 mN, to 3.9±0.5 mN after 10 min, to 3.6±0.4 mN after 15 min and to 3.5±0.4 mN after 20 min (**Fig. 2B**, left panel, ■). In the presence of both 0.03 mmol/l $BaCl_2$ and 0.01 mmol/l denatonium, the amplitudes of contractions were further reduced to 3.6±0.4 mN, 3.3±0.5 mN, 3.0±0.5 mN and to 2.9±0.4 mN after the same time intervals. Similar results of Ba^{2+} or Ba^{2+} and denatonium were obtained on the tetanic contractions.

All these data indicate that low concentrations of gentamicin or Ba^{2+} substantially reduce the inhibitory effect of denatonium on the EFS-induced single and tetanic contractions of abdominal skeletal muscles preparations *in vitro*.

Go to:

Discussion

To the best of our knowledge this is the first report on denatonium-dependent regulation of skeletal muscle function. The effective low concentration of denatonium suggests a selective denatonium-TAS2R interaction followed by a G-protein-dependent activation of PLC that breaks down PIP_2, into IP_3 and diacylglycerol (DAG), as well as weakens the EFS-induced contractions. This hypothesis is supported by the significantly suppressed effect of denatonium in the presence of gentamicin, the latter used to inhibit IP_3-formation (**Touchberry** *et al.* **2014**). It is known that application of higher concentrations of gentamicin can decrease the motor neuron stimulation of contraction because it is a competitive inhibitor of nAChR (**Amici** *et al.* **2005**) and thus it reduces the amplitudes of skeletal muscle contractions. However, under our experimental conditions, neuronal ACh mediation was eliminated and EFS stimulations excited only the skeletal muscles. Additionally, the low concentration of gentamicin greatly increased rather than suppressed the force of contractions in the presence of denatonium. Therefore, we assume that such a side effect is successfully avoided and almost a 'pure 'influence of gentamicin on $PIP_2/IP_3/DAG$-signaling is achieved. Also, the effective low concentration of gentamicin suggests that the influence of TAS2R activation on PIP_2 metabolism is not completely eliminated and this could be a reason for the partial block of denatonium-induced relaxation.

Another set of experiments targeted Kir channels. It is generally accepted that Kir2.1 and Kir2.2 channels are the prevalent forms of Kir channels in skeletal muscles (**DiFranco** *et al.* 2015). They are present either on the surface (about 30 %) or in T-tubules (about 70 %) of fibres (**DiFranco** *et al.* 2015). Kir channels play a crucial role in skeletal muscle excitability by keeping the extracellular concentration of K_+ low and thus the resting membrane potential at optimal value (**DiFranco** *et al.* 2015). Kir2.x channels are very important for keeping the physiological K_+ gradients, especially in T-tubules, because of the restricted intra T-tubular space that can be easily saturated by K_+ when K_+ return (influx) is disturbed. The latter will ultimately lead to membrane depolarization and will complicate the excitation-contraction coupling in the skeletal muscle fibres. Additionally, it is known that Kir2.1 channels has several PIP_2 binding sites which directly activate the channels (**Soom** *et al.* 2001). That is why, we tested Kir channel as possible participants in denatonium induced signaling using low concentration of $BaCl_2$ to block the channel. Similarly to gentamicin, barium ions reduced the effect of denatonium on the amplitudes of the studied contractions. These results suggest a link between Kir channels and TAS2R-induced reduction of amplitudes of single and tetanic contractions of rat abdominal muscles. Our data do not rule out the involvement of other cellular targets of the denatonium signal transduction pathway with significant effect on EFS-induced contractions.

The novel finding of our research is that denatonium regulates the contractility of rat abdominal skeletal muscle via TAS2R, PIP2 and its metabolites. This denatonium effect depends on the availability of Kir channels. Additionally, our study outlines the described preparations as an appropriate object of diverse physiological and pharmacological studies on TAS2R/PIP2/IP3+DAG signaling in skeletal muscles. The functional significance of IICR in them is still not very clear (Filip *et al.* 2019a, b), although all three IP3 receptor subtypes are expressed there, two of them ubiquitously (Santulli *et al.* 2017).

Phylogenetics of the Fascial System

Monitoring Editor: Alexander Muacevic and John R Adler
Leonardo Vieira⊠1
Author information Article notes Copyright and License information PMC Disclaimer

Go to:

Abstract

The fascial system, due to its enormous capacity to connect all other body systems, is currently highlighted for a better understanding of human life and health. The evolutionary theory is the most accepted explanation today to describe the development of this enormous variety of life on our planet. The report presents phylogenesis through the eyes of the fascial system. The development of the fascial system and its adaptations have made it possible to increase Homo sapiens' survival and success. We present a historical contextualization of the evolutionary theory followed by the main changes in the movement fasciae, in the transverse diaphragms, visceral fasciae, dermis, subcutaneous tissue, and neural fasciae. The article presents the evolutionary perspective with the resulting increase in efficiency with less energy expenditure.

Keywords: phylogenetic, fascial system, osteopathic medicine, fascia, physiotherapy

Go to:

Introduction and background

Charles Darwin, along with Alfred Wallace, proposed that all individuals came from a single ancestor. In his book, On the Origin of Species, published in 1858, Darwin impacted society at the time by presenting the theory of natural selection [1]. With the advancement of technology, some principles of this theory have undergone changes. The genetic revolution has also brought in new concepts and information about the evolutionary theory.

However, due to his importance in the field of evolutionary science, Darwin is considered the "father of evolution." According to Douglas Theobald, in a work published in 2010, the probability of all living beings having a single common ancestor is 102,860 times greater than the possibility of biological diversity having presented independent paths [2]. Hence, the evolutionary hypothesis has an enormous weight in the understanding of how we, Homo sapiens, have become the most adapted species on planet Earth.

Natural selection is a process composed of three common phenomena:

1) Principle of variation: every organism differs from others of the same species.

2) Genetic heredity: some variations present in all populations are inherited, transmitted genetically from parents to their children.

3) Differential reproductive success: all organisms, including humans, differ in the number of descendants they produce, which survive to reproduce.

Genetic modifications in individuals of a species that generate survival advantages increase reproductive chances and, consequently, generate more adapted descendants. The evolutionary process is stimulated mainly in times of scarcity. These advantages transmitted to the descendants and added to other acquisitions over many generations are passed on to an increasing group of individuals who, at any given moment, are no longer able to reproduce with the individuals of the old population. At this moment, a new species appears [3].

Basic precepts for life will always be taken into consideration to guide our discussion: the lower the energy expenditure, the greater the chance of survival (less allostatic load).

To make this possible, several adaptive events have occurred in all systems throughout the evolution of species. Few published works have explored the fascial system from an evolutionary perspective. The aim of this paper is to understand the importance of this system in the interaction with all the systems of the body and, at the same time, forming a link between all structures. The current definition of the fascial system as per the Fascia Research Society is as follows: "the fascial system consists of the three-dimensional continuum of soft, collagen-containing, loose and dense fibrous connective tissues that permeate the body. It incorporates elements such as adipose tissue, adventitia and neurovascular sheaths, aponeuroses, deep and superficial fasciae, epineurium, joint capsules, ligaments, membranes, meninges, myofascial expansions, periostea, retinacula, septa, tendons, visceral fasciae, and all the intramuscular and intermuscular connective tissues including endo-/peri-/epimysium. The fascial system surrounds, interweaves between, and interpenetrates all organs, muscles, bones, and nerve fibers, endowing the body with a functional structure, and providing an environment that enables all body systems to operate in an integrated manner" [4].

Knowledge about the phylogenesis of the fascial system would allow for a more productive assessment and intervention in promoting the individual's health. Although indivisible, we will use a didactic organizational segmentation used in several publications. We will divide this into four major topics: fasciae of movement, visceral fasciae, superficial fasciae, and neural fasciae.

Go to:

Review

Historical context

A major evolutionary milestone for sapiens was the use of the bipedal position for locomotion [5]. There is strong evidence to show that this advance was initiated at a time of major changes on our planet. Estimates indicate that between five and eight million years ago, there was a major climate change that affected the Earth. In East Africa, a forest-rich region, a great period of cooling changed the availability of natural resources. Until that fact, a great abundance of fruits and food had been available in those forests. This climatic change modified the entire local environmental structure, including the reduction of natural food resources for the great diversity of species that inhabited this region. There was high mortality of several species. Driven by the survival instinct, several species of animals left their natural environment to seek resources in other regions. Several of these species left in search of another location that would provide a greater chance of survival. Some species of animals reached the African savanna. Our emphasis will be given to the Homo genus to seek relations with our evolution.

In a more scarce environment, energy expenditure for locomotion in search of food becomes an important factor in natural selection. Some individuals of the Homo genus started to move in a bipedal position, of course not with the same skill as our current one. Measurements of energy expenditure show that bipedal stance actually consumes about four times less energy than quadrupedal stance in individuals with the same body weight [6]. Individuals who were able to travel long distances using less energy possibly obtained more food and increased their chance of survival. From several generations influenced by natural selection, a new species of individuals originated, our cousins in common with the chimpanzees, the Australopithecus, the first to use the bipedal position most of the time [7]. However, they presented great difficulties such as very flat feet, short legs, and rib cage shape still very similar to that of the chimpanzee. The gait still had a lot of lateral inclination, demanding a high energy expenditure compared to the human gait, but already much smaller than that of a chimpanzee [6]. These events bring a historical understanding to comprehend our phylogenetic adaptations. Chimpanzees are our closest living "cousins", with whom we share more than 98% of our genetic code [8]. From this point, we will generate a comparison in relation to the movement fasciae in order to understand our advantages.

Movement fasciae

Several musculoskeletal changes were necessary to adapt to the bipedal position. Skeletal changes such as changes in the shape of the bones of the foot, femur with enlarged valgus, enlargement of the pelvis, presence of a waist, and the appearance of another lumbar vertebra (Figure

(Figure1).
1). The organization of the spine in a curvature system with an inverted compensatory pattern was fundamental for changing the gravitational axis in the bipedal position [9].

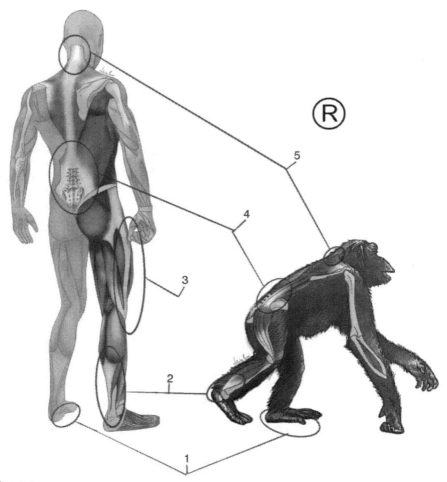

Figure 1
Phylogenetics of movement fasciae
1: plantar fascia; 2: Achilles tendon; 3: iliotibial band; 4: thoracolumbar fascia; 5 nuchal ligament

We present a plantar arch associated with an extremely efficient plantar fascia for transmitting force in relation to chimpanzees. When we walk, run, or jump, the plantar fascia takes advantage of the reaction force of the soil and transmits it upwards through the Achilles tendons [10]. Comparing the size of the human Achilles tendon with that of the chimpanzee, we observed a much larger tendon (Figure

(Figure1).
1). It is formed by the fascial expansions of the soleus, gastrocnemius, and plantar muscles [11]. In humans, the plantar muscle becomes less functional, and in some cases, it is not present at all. Also called the triceps surae tendon, it presents continuity with the posterior layer of the crural fascia [12]. Upon reaching the knee, a sophisticated center of fascial interaction, formed by retinacula, tendons, and ligaments, it transmits tension and modulates the support system, especially in the single-legged phase of gait.

An incredible variation of synovial bursae that interconnect, enabling great efficiency in protecting the joint and propagating the kinetic energy that ignites through the entire fascia lata, was formed by all the fasciae of the thigh [12]. The lateral part of the thigh is formed by a fibrous septum, the iliotibial tract, seen only in Homo sapiens, which leaves the lateral part of the tibia through the femur, where it is continuous with the fasciae of the gluteus maximus, gluteus medius, and tensor fascia lata (Figure

(Figure1). The
1). The iliotibial tract combined in its positional relationship with the gluteus fascia allowed to reduce the lateral trunk inclination in the single-legged support [13]. The gluteal fascia superiorly inserts itself into the thoracolumbar fascia, continuing the path of force transmission. The thoracolumbar fascia allows spine stabilization, control of the center of gravity, and synchronism between the pelvic and scapular girdle [14]. The thoracolumbar fascia is formed by the meeting of the fasciae of the abdominal muscles with those of the hip with the posterior torso. Its organization in the human species is so complex that we do not have a uniform anatomical classification. We will adopt the two-layer model mentioned by Willard et al. in 2012 [15].

We have an anterior and a posterior layer. The posterior part is subdivided into two compartments from the transverse process of the lumbar vertebrae: the most superficial layer of the posterior part, which is formed by the fascia of the gluteus maximus with the fascia of the reverse latissimus dorsi, acting on the control of movement mainly in the frontal and transverse planes. The deepest part of the posterior layer involves the erector muscles of the spine and the segmental muscles. In the lower region, it presents insertion in the periosteum of the sacrum, continuity with the sacrotuberous ligament, hamstring tendon, and fascia latae. Superiorly, it is continuous until the base of the skull. This region of the thoracolumbar fascia mainly controls movements in the sagittal plane, such as flexion-extension. In front of the transverse process, we have the anterior layer of the thoracolumbar fascia. This layer involves the psoas and quadratus lumborum muscles. Its adaptations allow an excellent ratio of the increased movements in the pelvis and trunk, especially those of extension. At the same time, this layer has an important relationship with the retroperitoneal organs, mainly the genitourinary system and the renal fascia [16]. Following the movement, the fascia of the trapezius muscle is continuous with the fascia of the latissimus dorsi, inserting itself superiorly into the entire nuchal ligament and also in the occipital bone [12] (Figure

(Figure1).
1). The nuchal ligament is a fascial junction of all the posterior fascial layers of the trunk linking all the cervical spine processes and the first two thoracic vertebrae [17]. This ligament interferes positively in the control of shear forces and in the formation of cervical lordosis generated by the new body alignment. In the upper cervical region, this ligament is continuous with the dura mater in the base of the skull [18]. Through this mechanism and all of the aforementioned chain, we can assume that the single-legged support can

function as a way of pumping by alternating tension in the region of the skull base through the connection of the nuchal ligament with the dura mater in that region. This mechanism possibly favors the maintenance of venous flow through the jugular foramen, keeping intracranial pressure stable during exhausting activities.

Bipedal stance allowed us to free our hands and upper limbs. This was important for us to develop great movements of the scapular girdle and limbs. The upper limb fasciae have a unique organization, allowing for a wide range and diversity of movements [13]. The upper limb is adapted to work in open kinetic chain movements, different from the reality presented by quadrupeds. As a consequence, the making of tools and the control of fire increased the chance of survival [3]. The complexity and efficiency of the tools increased as the skills and physical changes took place. This was accompanied by a great neurofascial organization giving an increasingly precise refinement to the distal movements of the upper limb [19]. The wrist left the quadrupedal flexion position for a wide variety of movements, allowing adjustments for fine movements [3]. An organization of the palmar fasciae into five independent layers associated with a large concentration of proprioceptive receptors in the retinacula on the wrist gives the sapiens precision [20].

The release of the scapular girdle for hunting movements, as a food uptake resource, was essential to increase the range of motion of the entire upper limb [21]. This gain in the release of the scapular waist, in addition to the refined coordination promoted by the thoracolumbar fascia, allowed great efficiency in handling the spear. This object allowed hunting at a distance, compensating for the sapiens 'decreased speed and, at the same time, decreasing the risk of corporal combat with prey, often infinitely stronger [3]. During a race, we have a great efficiency of this fascial system in the use of energy. The ankle retinacules are integrated in order to adjust to this demand, presenting a higher concentration of proprioceptors when compared to quadruped primates. In addition, the compartments of the feet assume a different configuration, giving up a gripping function, mainly by the hallux, for movements of extension and transmission of force in order to propel the body forward as a locomotion strategy [22].

Studies with kangaroos have shown a fundamental contribution of the fascial system to the efficiency of the locomotion movement [23]. When studying humans, the same power transmission capacity and kinetic energy savings demonstrated in gait, jump and run studies were proven. Kawakami et al., in 2002, demonstrated that at the moment of running in the deformation of the fascial system, the passive component was much larger than the musculoskeletal system, the active component. Even with great articular amplitudes, the movement occurred with the muscles contracting almost in an isometric way, while the fascial system presented great deformations, transmitting the force for the subsequent movements. This generates great energy savings through the mechanical and neuromuscular pathways [10].

In an analysis of the center of gravity, when jumping on unstable surfaces, it was demonstrated that a large part of the correction came from the passive component, generating great savings by decreasing the use of neuromuscular strategies [24]. The iliotibial tract stores about 7 joules of elastic energy per stride while running, saving energy for subsequent movements [25]. This also influences the strategy of maintaining the body without much oscillation in the single-legged support, since the corrections of inclinations of the body consume energy. The execution of eye movements in all directions and maintaining complete independence of the head and neck is an optimized feature in sapiens [26]. In addition to adaptations in the fascial system, through the Tenon capsule, there was an advanced neuromuscular control associated with changes in the eye structure itself [13-27].

The diaphragms

Our species is the only one that has five connective tissue structures anatomically arranged in a transversal form forming the five diaphragms of the body. They are, from cranial to caudal, as follows: the tentorium cerebelli, tongue (floor of the mouth), upper thoracic diaphragm, muscular diaphragm, and pelvic diaphragm (pelvis floor) [28]. These structures have a mechanical and neural connection, enabling several important functions for the bipedal position. They form limits of interdependent body cavities that, at the same time, need autonomy to perform various individual functions at different times. The five diaphragms provide us with control and synchronization of the intracavitary pressures, acting on the fluidic circulation between the cavities and also in the interstitium of the visceral parenchyma [28].

The tongue and floor of the mouth are innervated by five cranial pairs that direct their information to nuclei of the brain stem [29]. Mechanically it has continuity with all the fascias of the digestive tract and respiratory tract, reaching the base of the skull where it becomes continuous with the dura mater [30]. The upper thoracic diaphragm is formed by the upper portion of the endothoracic fascia and the junction of the parietal pleura with the deep layer of the deep fascia. It is innervated by the sympathetic spinal nerves. The new positional relationships of the clavicle, scapula, and shoulder promoted major adaptations. Only in sapiens does the junction between a movement fascia and a visceral fascia occur, forming the endothoracic fascia [31].

The diaphragm muscle in the quadrupeds helps in the movement of the torso laterality in locomotion. In sapiens, it plays an important role in synchronizing with the pelvic diaphragm, controlling the movements of the lower limb through the connection with the psoas muscle, in the new position, through the medial arcuate ligament [32]. The lumbar part helps to stabilize the lumbar region, especially in the second half of the forced expiration [33]. In quadrupeds, the diaphragm has a limited relationship with the pericardium and the heart. In bipeds, it starts to assume an important role in support, with greater influence on cardiac performance. It also plays an important role in tensioning the pharynx and larynx, participating in events such as speech and vomiting [34]. The action of reflux control by the diaphragm is enhanced in the bipedal position. The pelvic diaphragm is formed by the muscles and fasciae: ilium, ischium, and pubococcygeus, together with the piriformis fascia and obturator fascia being innervated by the sacral nerves [12]. Brainstem nuclei coordinate constant reflexes for synchronism, seeking to orchestrate the optimization of the body's functioning [28]. In the cranial fasciae session, we will detail the cerebellum tent more.

Visceral fasciae

The two systems that consume the most energy in the body are the digestive and the cerebral [3]. The primitive digestive system expends a lot of energy to break down food and make it usable for the body. Using strategies such as fermentation, lower mammals and even primates have organs such as voluminous large intestine (Figure

(Figure2).
2). A visceral fascial organization is automatically adapted to the new digestive demands [31].

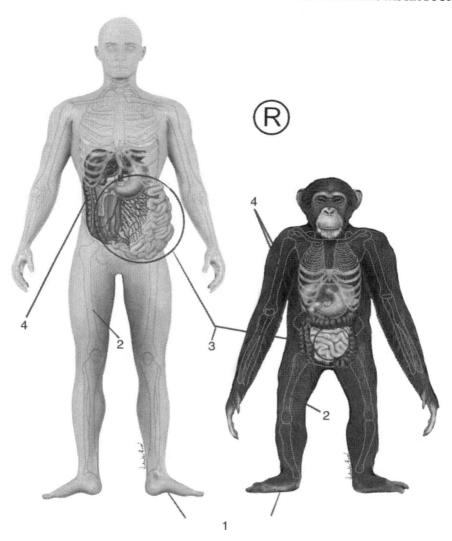

Figure 2
Phylogenetics of visceral fasciae
1: plantar fascia; 2: femur position; 3: small intestine and mesentery fascia; 4: large intestine

The effects of our ancestors 'experience on the African savanna environment resulted in major visceral changes. With food shortages, a great diversity of new foods was incorporated into the diet. The roots became a potential food with a lot of important nutrients [21]. At the same time, an increase in masticatory muscle mass and, automatically, a thickening of the respective fasciae of these muscles came as a consequence of the new demand. The connective tissue that forms the musculoskeletal structures on the face of mammals develops from the growth of the digestive system. The development of foregut releases gene factors responsible for attracting neural crest cells to form the connective tissue part of that region [35]. In response to the demand, individuals genetically stronger in their chewing presented an evolutionary advantage. This automatically reflects in a protrusion of the maxilla and mandible and consequently a retraction of the frontal part of the skull. As manual skills evolve, more powerful tools are manufactured [3].

The bipedal position changed the entire positioning relationship of the spine and viscera. With the horizontalization of the skull base, there is a change in the insertion axis of the buccopharyngeal fascia, changing the positioning and functioning of the nasopharynx, pharynx, hyoid bone, and larynx [26-30]. This alters the functional relationships in speech production, alters the spatial relationships for the development of the tongue and the hyoid, both in the digestive function and in the articulation of several different types of sounds. The relationship between tongue and epiglottis in sapiens is different from all other mammals. The space between the base of the tongue and the soft palate is greater in sapiens [26].

We have a lower and shorter larynx compared to other primates. Our babies have a high, nasal larynx, like most adult mammals, favoring gas exchange in the first months of life. In addition, human babies have a limited degree of neuromuscular control. The intracranial larynx decreases the risk of aspirating milk or saliva. By the third month, the larynx is already in a lower position. The rapid growth of the mandibular and maxillary arches together with the development of the skull and cervical base, associated with the development of the digestive and respiratory systems, results in a repositioning of the larynx, located below the hyoid [26]. The middle layer of the deep cervical fascia together with the fasciae of the mandible, the floor of the mouth and tongue are remodeled to the new positioning, and also to the new functions. A smaller tongue, however, as well as movements and a very efficient sensory and muscular system increased the variety of possibilities. The tongue is continuous with visceral fasciae that follow the digestive tract inferiorly and also superiorly to the base of the skull [30]. In this region, the connective tissue continues with the dura mater that surrounds the foramen of the passage of the vessels that penetrate the skull [36]. It also has continuity with the visceral fasciae of the respiratory tube and larynx, providing extremely diverse sound production. The angle between the nasopharynx and the respiratory tube is close to 90 degrees and with the acquisition of the external nose turned downwards, associated with a peculiar arrangement of the nasal conchae of the internal nose, creating a favorable environment for humidification and heating of the air, and enabling greater efficiency in gas exchange at the pulmonary level. At the same time, due to this disposition, during great efforts, where the breathing becomes more intense, there is a considerable increase in the flow and this starts to have a turbulent trajectory. This allows a much larger amount of air to have more contact with the surface of the nasal mucosa and consequently a greater concentration of air that reaches the alveoli with the potential to be captured [26].

At the cervical level, we have a new organization of the middle layer of the deep fascia, also known as pretracheal fascia. This fascia is formed by two laminae: the first and most superficial involves the infrahyoid muscles and is important for the new mechanisms of language and the deglutition relationship of the bipedal posture. The deepest lamina surrounds the thyroid and the parathyroid presenting continuity with the pericardium, forming the suspensory ligaments of the pericardium [36]. This structure is important due to gravity. In addition, the thyroid has undergone important developments to adjust to the new metabolic demand and its role is fundamental in the circadian rhythm. Its hormones act on metabolism and also on the pineal gland influencing tissue replacement in the body [37].

The bipedal position has important consequences for the development of visceral fasciae. A very important phylogenetic adaptation in sapiens is the change in the relationship between the parietal lung pleura and the fasciae of the trunk. In lower mammals, when moving around at a speed, they use the respiratory strategy always linked to the positioning of limbs and thorax. In the high-speed phase when they reach trunk extension and maximum limb distance, the inspiratory moment occurs, and the expiratory moment occurs at the moment of trunk flexion with the approach of the limbs [3]. Despite the efficiency from the speed point of view, this respiratory link to musculoskeletal movements prevents the strategy of gasp, which constitutes an efficient internal cooling mechanism. When moving at high speed for a long time, the internal organs overheat, causing the system to collapse. In sapiens, the parietal pleura merges with the deep intercostal fascia. This allows the independence of the respiratory moment with the movement of the trunk and limbs. At the same time that the sapiens lose speed jogging, the ability to run for longer distances increases. This all adds up to refrigeration strategies promoted by changes in the superficial fasciae and dermis, as we will see in the respective section of this article. The independence of breathing in relation to the movement system and phonation allows greater efficiency in all of these systems.

Bipedalism brought about refinement to the movements of the

upper limbs. As a result of this came the dominance of fire and the improvement of hunting tools, bringing significant changes in hunting and in the conditions for preparing food. Large animals, protein, and animal fat brought important energy subsidies to new demands. Owing to this, our ancestors started to use the masticatory apparatus much less, because the food became much softer [3]. This caused a decrease in the size of the muscles and fasciae of the masticatory apparatus. A consequent retraction of the viscerocranium, maxilla, and mandible gave space for the frontal region, the neurocranium, to evolve. Digestive strategies, such as fermentation, became less important in the body. The large intestine decreased its size and there was an increase in the size of the small intestine and consequently a larger area for nutrient absorption (Figure

(Figure2)
2) [38]. The increased food diversity also generated an increase in the number of microorganisms establishing a symbiotic relationship in the small intestine, because, in addition to helping with digestion, they released several important substances that acted in the development of the brain [39]. With all this, the energy balance underwent major changes. Less energy was spent on digestion, more nutrients were absorbed by the system. The frontal region now had a greater possibility of growth and available energy for this to occur [3].

Important changes have also occurred in the pelvic visceral fasciae. The action of gravity in the bipedal position and the increase in the width of the pelvis changed visceral relations, and especially of the organs and fasciae of the smaller pelvis. The increased lateral diameter minimized the pressure effect of the bipedal position [3]. In addition, changes occurred in the suspensory ligaments of pelvic organs. Substantial changes occurred at the level of the pelvic diaphragm in order to sustain the imposed demand. At that moment, a dissipation of force by the intravisceral movements between the insertional fasciae, which constitutes each outermost visceral fascial, was able to minimize gravitational effects. For this, sapiens had an increase in loose connective tissue and intravisceral fat. An increase in the size of the small intestine associated with a bipedal position generated important changes in the mesentery. The visceral fascia that surrounds the jejunum and ileum was adjusted to adapt to a considerable increase in the vascular network for a greater intake of nutrients [31-38].

Dermis and subcutaneous tissue

The dermis and subcutaneous tissue are part of a large fascial system that involves the entire body [4]. Major acquisitions in the dermis and subcutaneous tissue have become fundamental to the adaptive success of sapiens [40].

The dermis is the layer located just below the epidermis, participating in the constitution of the skin. It represents the most innervated fascial tissue in the human body. It presents high concentrations of primitive, polymodal neural receptors, very simple in their physical constitution [41]. These receptors are called interceptors that control the conditions of the body's internal environment, informing the central nervous system of various types of information including nociceptive [42]. The great evolution of sapiens is the destination of this information. The information travels from the skin to the posterior horn of the spinal cord, making the first synapse ascending to the upper centers, with the final destination being the insular cortex. The soft dermal touch promotes a feeling of pleasure and well-being in the mammals related to conviviality and interaction. These interactions are even stronger in Homo sapiens. Human beings have reached the peak of social interactions, greatly increasing the chance of survival. This type of sensation promoted by light touch is also called sensual touch and also promotes the stimulation of higher centers linked to sexuality [43]. These two acquisitions meet the two laws of the evolutionary principle: survival and reproduction. They also have a large concentration of phylogenetically more evolved receptors, encapsulated, and with the presence of fat in their composition, such as Meissner, Merkel, Pacini, and Ruffini [44]. This was very important in the proprioceptive and exteroceptive refinement, managing to improve the positioning relationships of the body in space and the perceptions of the external environment.

In the sapiens dermis, there is an average of 5-10 million sweat glands spread throughout the body and which constitute an efficient cooling system, which we will explain below [3]. Primates have sweat glands in specific areas of the body such as the feet, hands, and genitals. The subcutaneous tissue is basically composed of two layers of fat separated by a layer of loose connective tissue, the superficial fascia itself. The most superficial layer of fat establishes a direct relationship with the dermis. It presents an organized collagen network arranged perpendicularly to the skin, with the optimized function in the matter of impact cushioning. The deepest layer of fat has a direct relationship with the deep layer of the deep fascia, which is the first layer of movement. It presents an organization of collagen with an oblique disposition favoring the sliding between the layers, mitigating the effects of muscle contraction and movement fasciae on the most superficial layers [12].

The subcutaneous tissue layer, in addition to being richly innervated, has a vast vascular network. About 70% of the body's lymphatic and venous network is in this tissue [31]. The interaction between this tissue and the dermis promotes a great survival advantage for sapiens in relation to all other animals. In exhaustive physical activities or in very hot climatic conditions, such as in African savannas, a large amount of sweat produced by the dermal sweat glands is spread throughout the body, including the head region. When sweat comes into contact with air, it cools the skin. This has a cooling effect on the large blood circulation in the superficial veins of the subcutaneous tissue. This blood flows throughout the body, cooling the organs and also the brain. This mechanism is essential for maintaining extreme conditions, preventing the internal system from collapsing due to overheating [26]. This advantage was fundamental to our hunter-gathering ancestors. Bipedal running is less efficient in terms of speed than sprinting. However, when moving at speed, the quadrupeds are unable to use their main cooling mechanism, the gasping. As a result, our ancestors chased prey until their system collapsed due to overheating. Hence they were easily slaughtered [21]. In the cerebral part, there were other adaptations that we will highlight in the section on the evolution of the cranial fasciae.

Sapiens presents a mimic musculature with a great diversity of movements, an important evolutionary development for social organization. In the face region, we have a junction of the superficial fascia with the movement fascia [12].

Neural fasciae

The advent of the bipedal position brought about several changes in the fascial system of the human head and cervical spine, maintaining the horizontality of the look and, at the same time, adequate stability of the skull and cervical joint. The occipital condyles are designed to allow a very little movement. Strong ligament complexes are incorporated into the region [26]. Important relationships, already present in primates, have been refined, such as, for example, the connection with the dura mater at the base of the skull. The fascia of the occipital muscles and the nuchal ligament have direct insertions in the dura mater in the upper cervical [45]. In the frontal region of the skull, the epicranial fascia interconnects the base of the skull with the Tenon capsule, in the orbital region. The Tenon capsule is continuous with the cranial dura mater, allowing direct mechanical coordination between the base and the eye region [27]. These connections facilitate the synchronism and, at the same time, the independence of the movements of the head with the movements of the eyeball. In addition, sapiens present a high concentration of proprioceptive receptors in the muscular fasciae, mainly in the perimysium of the suboccipital muscles [46]. This neurofascial interaction allows for a refined synchronization of skull control during postural demands and movement.

Studies of head development analysis demonstrate that the development of the anterior part of the cortex, especially the frontal cortex, is stimulated by gene factors released from the development of the digestive tract [35]. It is likely that the evolution of sapiens 'foregut in the bipedal position directly influenced the great cortical evolution of our species. This demonstrates the difficulty of segmenting human systems because, in reality, the development of one structure directly or indirectly influences the development of another, even though they belong to different systems. The cerebral cortex shows an enormous growth in the sapiens, practically doubling in relation to the chimpanzee (Figure

(Figure3).
3). There was a great growth of the frontal and prefrontal cortex, with the acquisition of nuclei, which allowed the capacity for deep conscious analysis, a great capacity for abstraction, future projections, and increasingly organized social interactions. Broca's and Wernicke's areas present a large increase in volume in relation to primates allowing a great evolution of the language and communication system in general [26-37].

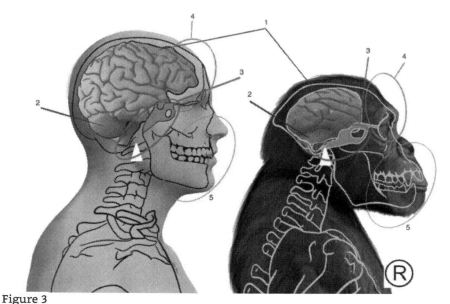

Figure 3
Comparison between the human cortex and the chimpanzee cortex
1: cortex; 2: cerebellum; 3: relationship of sphenoid with foramen magnum; 4: frontal cortex; 5: maxilla and mandible

In the anterior region of the skull, the retraction of the visceral cranium was accompanied by a protrusion of the frontal region. This promoted a change in the angles of the sphenobasilar synchondrosis and in the angle between the orbit and the cranial base (Figure

(Figure3).
3). Consequently, the organization of the dural compartments has also undergone changes [26]. The tension lines of the falx of the brain, formed by the upper part of the dura mater altered its conformation due to the change in the position of the ethmoid and consequently the crista galli, where the falx is inserted. The falx of the brain subsequently converges to the internal occipital protuberance. In mammals, this region has a more posterior location in relation to primates due to the greater development of cortical, cerebellar areas, and changes in the development of

the squamous part of the occipital bone (Figure

(Figure3)
3) [47]. The region of the internal occipital protuberance also receives the insertion of the cerebellum falx, which divides and organizes the cerebellum into two hemispheres at a horizontal level. At the horizontal level, the change in the organization of the sphenoid promotes a change in the diaphragm of the sella turcica, which represents one of the parts formed by the invagination of the meningeal dura mater, where the pituitary is located. The tentorium cerebelli represents the fourth dural organization [34]. It presents a horizontal arrangement fixing laterally on the petrous crests of the temporal, previously on the lower wings of the sphenoid, more precisely in the anterior clinoid processes. It follows posteriorly around the edge of the posterior cranial fossa bilaterally, meeting in the internal occipital protuberance, at the border between the endochondral part and the intramembranous part of the occipital bone. Its structure is greatly modified in sapiens to support the large increase in cortical weight in conjunction with the change in the center of gravity. Part of this support is given by the other parts of the dura mater that present continuity, distributing the stresses to all pillars through the organization of collagen fibers forming dural bands of force transmission [18].

The dura mater actively participates in regulating the ossification of the bones at the apex of the head. The region of the sagittal and coronal sutures is where the greatest growth occurs in sapiens. Dura mater acts as a mediator in the relationship between very high brain growth and the rapid development of the bones of the cranial vault [47]. This dural adaptation allowed greater efficiency in the shape and function of the venous sinuses. The confluence of the sinuses became more superior, together with the straight sinus, increasing the efficiency of the brain's cranial drainage system [48].

At the peripheral level, with the increase in the possibility of movement, the mechanical interfaces between the peripheral nerves and the tissues to which they pass have also undergone modifications. The mesoneurium, made up of loose connective tissue, is reinforced in places of greater mobility. A greater number of receptors and more specific ones have been incorporated, mainly in the joint tissue, to organize increasingly complex movements and tension lines. At the medullary level, increasingly sophisticated modulation processes were generating several adjustments in the conjunctive system without the participation of the cortex [19].

At the brainstem level, synchronized control between body systems has been incorporated in addition to the possibility of isolated actions of various systems, greatly increasing the possibility of functioning by peripheral control [19]. At this level, modulatory reactions have been improved, preventing various information from being processed by the brain, generating great energy savings. A great evolution in neuronal nuclei such as the ambiguous nucleus allowed a greater possibility of facial expressions, together with the control of cervical movements and refinement in pressure control. This nucleus coordinates information regarding the nerves: vagus, spinal accessory, glossopharyngeal, and facial [49]. The cerebellum holds about 80% of the brain's neuronal bodies, refining control and motor coordination, helping to refine existing movements at the same time and allowing the execution of increasingly complex movements [50].

The ligaments between the medulla and the medullary canal were remodeled in relation to the new demand. The curvatures of the spine modified the relations of the medulla and meninges with the medullary canal. Adaptations in the anterior ligaments, such as the yellow and anterior longitudinal, were necessary in order to allow an increase in mobility of the spine, especially in the extension movement. At the cranial level, major changes occurred allowing adaptations for cortical growth and organization of brain areas. Although the region of the base of the skull is considered to be older from a phylogenetic point of view, the horizontalization of the foramen magnum greatly changed the meningeal relations of the region, providing an organization that promotes stability and functionality in the high cervical transition and brain bulb. The occipital bone is formed by mesodermal cells from the first four somites, called occipital somites [26].

Go to:

Conclusions

The fascial system, due to its function of interconnecting all the systems of the body, has great importance in the mechanism of operation and energy saving. Understanding the phylogenetic evolution of this system allows us to expand the possibilities of identifying dysfunctional zones responsible for the increase in energy expenditure leading to an increase in the allostatic load and, consequently, assuming pathologies. The evolutionary knowledge of the fascial system allows us to design conducts in order to optimize the characteristics that make human beings the most adapted species on the planet. We hope that this study will provide a stimulus to researchers to seek further clarifications regarding the evolutionary processes of the fascial system, especially given the scarcity of publications on the subject.

Hyaluronan and synovial joint: function, distribution and healing

Tamer Mahmoud Tamer[1,2]

Author information Article notes Copyright and License information PMC Disclaimer

Go to:

Abstract

Synovial fluid is a viscous solution found in the cavities of synovial joints. The principal role of synovial fluid is to reduce friction between the articular cartilages of synovial joints during movement. The presence of high molar mass hyaluronan (HA) in this fluid gives it the required viscosity for its function as lubricant solution. Inflammation oxidation stress enhances normal degradation of hyaluronan causing several diseases related to joints.

This review describes hyaluronan properties and distribution, applications and its function in synovial joints, with short review for using thiol compounds as antioxidants preventing HA degradations under inflammation conditions.

Keywords: synovial joint fluid, hyaluronan, antioxidant, thiol compound

Go to:

Introduction

The human skeleton consists of both fused and individual bones supported and supplemented by ligaments, tendons, and skeletal muscles. Articular ligaments and tendons are the main parts holding together the joint(s). In respect of movement, there are freely moveable, partially moveable, and immovable joints. Synovial joints (**Figure 1**), the freely moveable ones, allow for a large range of motion and encompass wrists, knees, ankles, shoulders, and hips (Kogan, 2010).

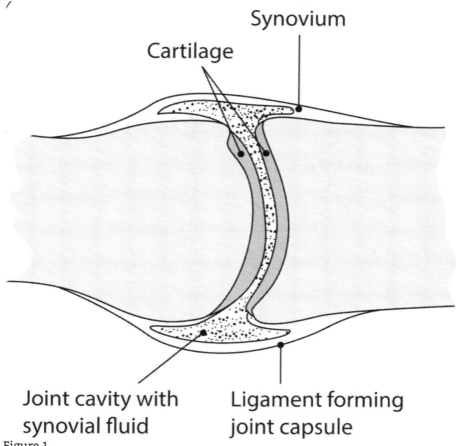

Cartilage

Synovium

Joint cavity with synovial fluid

Ligament forming joint capsule

Figure 1
Normal, healthy synovial joint (adapted from Kogan, 2010).

Go to:

Structure of synovial joints

Cartilage

In a healthy synovial joint, heads of the bones are encased in a smooth (hyaline) cartilage layer. These tough slippery layers – *e.g.* those covering the bone ends in the knee joint – belong to mechanically highly stressed tissues in the human body. At walking, running, or sprinting the strokes frequency attain approximately 0.5, 2.5 or up to 10 Hz.

Cartilage functions also as a shock absorber. This property is derived from its high water entrapping capacity as well as from the structure and intermolecular interactions among polymeric components that constitute the cartilage tissue (Servaty *et al.*, 2000). Figure 2 sketches a section of the cartilage – a chondrocyte cell that permanently restructures/rebuilds its extracellular matrix. Three classes of proteins exist in articular cartilage: collagens (mostly type II collagen); proteoglycans (primarily aggrecan); and other noncollagenous proteins (including link protein, fibronectin, COMP – cartilage oligomeric matrix protein) and the smaller proteoglycans (biglycan, decorin, and fibromodulin). The interaction between highly negatively charged cartilage proteoglycans and type II collagen fibrils is responsible for the compressive and tensile strength of the tissue, which resists applied load *in vivo*.

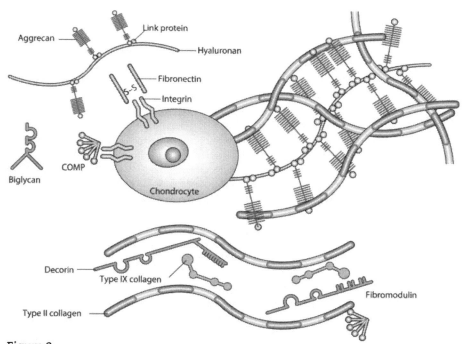

Figure 2
Articular cartilage main components and structure (adapted from Chen *et al.*, 2006).

Synovium/synovial membrane

Each synovial joint is surrounded by a fibrous, highly vascular capsule/envelope called synovium, whose internal surface layer is lined with a synovial membrane. Inside this membrane, type B synoviocytes (fibroblast-like cell lines) are localized/embedded. Their primary function is to continuously extrude high-molar-mass hyaluronans (HAs) into synovial fluid.

Synovial fluid

The synovial fluid (SF) of natural joints normally functions as a biological lubricant as well as a biochemical pool through which nutrients and regulatory cytokines traverse. SF contains molecules that provide low-friction and low-wear properties to articulating cartilage surfaces.

Molecules postulated to play a key role in lubrication alone or in combination, are proteoglycan 4 (PRG4) (Swann *et al.*, 1985) present in SF at a concentration of 0.05–0.35 mg/ml (Schmid *et al.*, 2001), hyaluronan (HA) (Ogston & Stanier, 1953) at 1–4 mg/ml (Mazzucco *et al.*, 2004), and surface-active phospholipids (SAPL) (Schwarz & Hills, 1998) at 0.1 mg/ml (Mazzucco *et al.*, 2004). Synoviocytes secrete PRG4 (Jay *et al.*, 2000; Schumacher *et al.*, 1999) and are the major source of SAPL (Dobbie *et al.*, 1995; Hills & Crawford, 2003; Schwarz & Hills, 1996), as well as HA (Haubeck *et al.*, 1995; Momberger *et al.*, 2005) in SF. Other cells also secrete PRG4, including chondrocytes in the superficial layer of articular cartilage (Schmid *et al.*, 2001b; Schumacher *et al.*, 1994) and, to a much lesser extent, cells in the meniscus (Schumacher *et al.*, 2005).

As a biochemical depot, SF is an ultra filtrate of blood plasma that is concentrated by virtue of its filtration through the synovial membrane. The synovium is a thin lining (~ 50 µm in humans) comprised of tissue macrophage A cells, fibroblast-like

B cells (Athanasou & Quinn, 1991; Revell, 1989; Wilkinson *et al.*, 1992), and fenestrated capillaries (Knight & Levick, 1984). It is backed by a thicker layer (~ 100 μm) of loose connective tissue called the subsynovium (SUB) that includes an extensive system of lymphatics for clearance of transported molecules. The cells in the synovium form a discontinuous layer separated by intercellular gaps of several microns in width (Knight & Levick, 1984; McDonald & Levick, 1988). The extracellular matrix in these gaps contains collagen types I, III, and V (Ashhurst *et al.*, 1991; Rittig *et al.*, 1992), hyaluronan (Worrall *et al.*, 1991), chondroitin sulphate (Price *et al.*, 1996; Worrall *et al.*, 1994), biglycan and decorin proteoglycans (Coleman *et al.*, 1998), and fibronectin (Poli *et al.*, 2004). The synovial matrix provides the permeable pathway through which exchange of molecules occurs (Levick, 1994), but also offers sufficient outflow resistance (Coleman *et al.*, 1998; Scott *et al.*, 1998) to retain large solutes of SF within the joint cavity. Together, the appropriate reflection of secreted lubricants by the synovial membrane and the appropriate lubricant secretion by cells are necessary for development of a mechanically functional SF (Blewis *et al.*, 2007).

In the joint, HA plays an important role in the protection of articular cartilage and the transport of nutrients to cartilage. In patients with rheumatoid arthritis (RA), (**Figure 3**) it has been reported that HA acts as an anti inflammatory substance by inhibiting the adherence of immune complexes to neutrophils through the Fc receptor (Brandt, 1970), or by protecting the synovial tissues from the attachment of inflammatory mediators (Miyazaki *et al.*, 1983, Mendichi & Soltes, 2002).

NORMAL JOINT

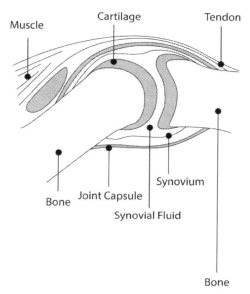

JOINT AFFECTED BY RHEUMATOID ARTHRITIS

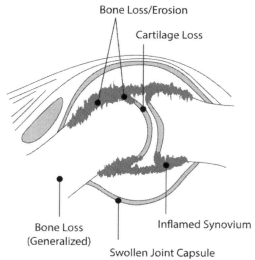

Figure 3

Normal, (healthy) and rheumatoid arthritis synovial joint.

Reactive oxygen species (ROS) ($O_2 \cdot^-$, H_2O_2, $\cdot OH$) are generated in abundance by synovial neutrophils from RA patients, as compared with synovial neutrophils of osteoarthritis (OA) patients and peripheral neutrophils of both RA and OA patients (Niwa *et al.*, 1983).

McCord (1973) demonstrated that HA was susceptible to degradation by ROS *In vitro*, and that this could be protected by superoxide dismutase (SOD) and/or catalase, which suggests the possibility that there is pathologic oxidative damage to synovial fluid components in RA patients. Dahl *et al.* (1985) reported that there are reduced HA concentrations in synovial fluids from RA patients. It has also been reported that ROS scavengers inhibit the degradation of HA by ROS (Soltes, 2010; Blake *et al.*, 1981; Betts & Cleland, 1982; Soltes *et al.*, 2004).

These findings appear to support the hypothesis that ROS are responsible for the accelerated degradation of HA in the rheumatoid joint. In the study of Juranek and Soltes (2012) the oxygen radical scavenging activities of synovial fluids from both RA and OA patients were assessed, and the antioxidant activities of these synovial fluids were analyzed by separately examining HA, d-glucuronic acid, and *N*-acetyl-d-glucosamine.

Go to:

Hyaluronan

In 1934, Karl Meyer and his colleague John Palmer isolated a previously unknown chemical substance from the vitreous body of cows 'eyes. They found that the substance contained two sugar molecules, one of which was uronic acid. For convenience, therefore, they proposed the name "hyaluronic acid". The popular name is derived from "hyalos", which is the Greek word for glass + uronic acid (Meyer & Palmer, 1934). At the time, they did not know that the substance which they had discovered would prove to be one of the most interesting and useful natural macromolecules. HA was first used commercially in 1942 when Endre Balazs applied for a patent to use it as a substitute for egg white in bakery products (Necas *et al.*, 2008).

The term "hyaluronan" was introduced in 1986 to conform to the international nomenclature of polysaccharides and is attributed to Endre Balazs (Balazs *et al.,* 1986) who coined it to encompass the different forms the molecule can take, e.g, the acid form, hyaluronic acid, and the salts, such as sodium hyaluronate, which forms at physiological pH (Laurent, 1989). HA was subsequently isolated from many other sources and the physicochemical structure properties and biological role of this polysaccharide were studied in numerous laboratories (Kreil, 1995). This work has been summarized in a Ciba Foundation Symposium (Laurent, 1989) and a recent review (Laurent & Fraser, 1992; Chabrecek *et al.,* 1990; Orvisky *et al.,* 1992).

Hyaluronan (**Figure** 4) is a unique biopolymer composed of repeating disaccharide units formed by *N*-acetyl-d-glucosamine and d-glucuronic acid. Both sugars are spatially related to glucose which in the β-configuration allows all of its bulky groups (the hydroxyls, the carboxylate moiety, and the anomeric carbon on the adjacent sugar) to be in sterically favorable equatorial positions while all of the small hydrogen atoms occupy the less sterically favorable axial positions. Thus, the structure of the disaccharide is energetically very stable. HA is also unique in its size, reaching up to several million Daltons and is synthesized at the plasma membrane rather than in the Golgi, where sulfated glycosaminoglycans are added to protein cores (Itano & Kimata, 2002; Weigel *et al.,* 1997; Kogan *et al.,* 2007a).

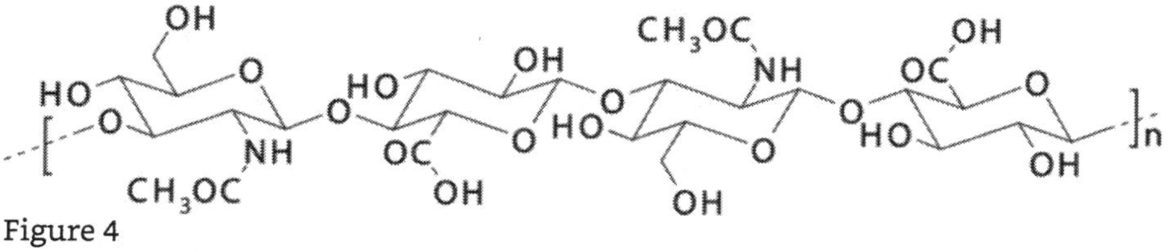

Figure 4

Structural formula of hyaluronan – the acid form.

In a physiological solution, the backbone of a HA molecule

is stiffened by a combination of the chemical structure of the disaccharide, internal hydrogen bonds, and interactions with the solvent. The axial hydrogen atoms form a non-polar, relatively hydrophobic face while the equatorial side chains form a more polar, hydrophilic face, thereby creating a twisting ribbon structure. Solutions of hyaluronan manifest very unusual rheological properties and are exceedingly lubricious and very hydrophilic. In solution, the hyaluronan polymer chain takes on the form of an expanded, random coil. These chains entangle with each other at very low concentrations, which may contribute to the unusual rheological properties. At higher concentrations, solutions have an extremely high but shear-dependent viscosity. A 1% solution is like jelly, but when it is put under pressure it moves easily and can be administered through a small-bore needle. It has therefore been called a "pseudo-plastic" material. The extraordinary rheological properties of hyaluronan solutions make them ideal as lubricants. There is evidence that hyaluronan separates most tissue surfaces that slide along each other. The extremely lubricious properties of hyaluronan have been shown to reduce postoperative adhesion formation following abdominal and orthopedic surgery. As mentioned, the polymer in solution assumes a stiffened helical configuration, which can be attributed to hydrogen bonding between the hydroxyl groups along the chain. As a result, a coil structure is formed that traps approximately 1000 times its weight in water (Chabrecek *et al.*, 1990; Cowman & Matsuoka, 2005; Schiller *et al.*, 2011)

Go to:

Properties of hyaluronan

Hyaluronan networks

The physico-chemical properties of hyaluronan were studied in detail from 1950 onwards (Comper & Laurent, 1978).

The molecules behave in solution as highly hydrated randomly kinked coils, which start to entangle at concentrations of less than 1 mg/mL. The entanglement point can be seen both by sedimentation analysis (Laurent *et al.*, 1960) and viscosity (Morris *et al.*, 1980). More recently Scott and his group have given evidence that the chains when entangling also interact with each other and form stretches of double helices so that the network becomes mechanically more firm (Scott *et al.*, 1991).

Rheological properties

Solutions of hyaluronan are viscoelastic and the viscosity is markedly shearing dependent (Morris *et al.*, 1980; Gibbs *et al.*, 1968). Above the entanglement point the viscosity increases rapidly and exponentially with concentration ($\sim c_{3.3}$) (Morris *et al.*, 1980) and a solution of 10 g/l may have a viscosity at low shear of $\sim 10_6$ times the viscosity of the solvent. At high shear the viscosity may drop as much as $\sim 10_3$ times (Gibbs *et al.*, 1968). The elasticity of the system increases with increasing molecular weight and concentration of hyaluronan as expected for a molecular network. The rheological properties of hyaluronan have been connected with lubrication of joints and tissues and hyaluronan is commonly found in the body between surfaces that move along each other, for example cartilage surfaces and muscle bundles (Bothner & Wik, 1987).

Water homeostasis

A fixed polysaccharide network offers a high resistance to bulk flow of solvent (Comper & Laurent, 1978). This was demonstrated by Day (1950) who showed that hyaluronidase treatment removes a strong hindrance to water flow through a fascia. Thus HA and other polysaccharides prevent excessive fluid fluxes through tissue compartments. Furthermore, the osmotic pressure of a hyaluronan solution is non-ideal and increases exponentially with the concentration. In spite of the high molecular weight of the polymer the osmotic pressure of a 10 g/l hyaluronan solution is of the same order as an l0 g/l albumin solution. The exponential relationship makes hyaluronan and other polysaccharides excellent osmotic buffering substances – moderate changes in concentration lead to marked changes in osmotic pressure. Flow resistance together with osmotic buffering makes hyaluronan an ideal regulator of the water homeostasis in the body.

Network interactions with other macromolecules

The hyaluronan network retards the diffusion of other molecules (Comper & Laurent, 1978; Simkovic *et al.*, 2000). It can be shown that it is the steric hindrance which restricts the movements and not the viscosity of the solution. The larger the molecule the more it will be hindered. *In vivo* hyaluronan will therefore act as a diffusion barrier and regulate the transport of other substances through the intercellular spaces. Furthermore, the network will exclude a certain volume of solvent for other molecules; the larger the molecule the less space will be available to it (Comper & Laurent, 1978). A solution of 10 g/l of hyaluronan will exclude about half of the solvent to serum albumin. Hyaluronan and other polysaccharides therefore take part in the partition of plasma proteins between the vascular and extravascular spaces. The excluded volume phenomenon will also affect the solubility of other macromolecules in the interstitium, change chemical equilibria and stabilize the structure of, for example, collagen fibers.

Medical applications of hyaluronic acid

The viscoelastic matrix of HA can act as a strong biocompatible support material and is therefore commonly used as growth scaffold in surgery, wound healing and embryology. In addition, administration of purified high molecular weight HA into orthopaedic joints can restore the desirable rheological properties and alleviate some of the symptoms of osteoarthritis (Balazs & Denlinger, 1993; Balazs & Denlinger, 1989; Kogan *et al.*, 2007). The success of the medical applications of HA has led to the production of several successful commercial products, which have been extensively reviewed previously.

Table 1 summarizes both the medical applications and the commonly used commercial preparations containing HA used within this field. HA has also been extensively studied in ophthalmic, nasal and parenteral drug delivery. In addition, more novel applications including pulmonary, implantation and gene delivery have also been suggested. Generally, HA is thought to act as either a mucoadhesive and retain the drug at its site of action/absorption or to modify the *in vivo* release/absorption rate of the therapeutic agent. A summary of the drug delivery applications of HA is shown in Table 2.

Table 1

Summary of the medical applications of hyaluronic acid (Brown & Jones, 2005).

Disease state	Applications	Commercial products	Publications
Osteoarthritis	Lubrication and mechanical support for the joints	Hyalgan® (Fidia, Italy) Artz® (Seikagaku, Japan) ORTHOVISC® (Anika, USA) Healon®, Opegan® and Opelead®	Hochburg, 2000; Altman, 2000; Dougados, 2000; Guidolin *et al.*, 2001; Maheu *et al.*, 2002; Barrett & Siviero, 2002; Miltner *et al.*, 2002;Tascioglu and Oner, 2003; Uthman *et al.*, 2003; Kelly *et al.*, 2003; Hamburger *et al.*, 2003; Kirwan, 2001; Ghosh & Guidolin, 2002; Mabuchi *et*

			al., 1999; Balazs, 2003; Fraser *et al.,* 1993; Zhu & Granick, 2003.
Surgery and wound healing	Implantation of artificial intraocular lens, viscoelastic gel	Bionect®, Connettivina® and Jossalind®	Ghosh & Jassal, 2002; Risbert, 1997; Inoue & Katakami, 1993; Miyazaki *et al.,* 1996; Stiebel-Kalish *et al.,* 1998; Tani *et al.,* 2002; Vazquez *et al.,* 2003; Soldati *et al.,* 1999; Ortonne, 1996; Cantor *et al.,* 1998; Turino & Cantor, 2003.
Embryo implantation	Culture media for the use of *In vitro* fertilizatio n	EmbryoGlue® (Vitrolife, USA)	Simon *et al.,* 2003; Gardner *et al.,* 1999; Vanos *et al.,* 1991; Kemmann, 1998; Suchanek *et al.,* 1994; Joly *et al.,* 1992; Gardner, 2003; Lane *et al.,* 2003; Figueiredo *et al.,* 2002, Miyano *et al.,* 1994; Kano *et al.,* 1998; Abeydeera, 2002; Jaakma *et al.,* 1997; Furnus *et al.,* 1998; Jang *et al.,* 2003.

Open in a separate window

Table 2

Summary of the drug delivery applications of hyaluronic acid.

Route	Justification	Therapeutic agents	Publications

Ophthalmic	Increased ocular residence of drug, which can lead to increased bioavailability	Pilocarpine, tropicamide, timolol, gentimycin, tobramycin,arecaidine polyester, (S) aceclidine	Jarvinen *et al.*, 1995; Sasaki *et al.*, 1996; Gurny *et al.*, 1987; Camber *et al.*, 1987; Camber & Edman, 1989; Saettone *et al.*, 1994; Saettone *et al.*, 1991; Bucolo *et al.*, 1998; Bucolo & Mangiafico, 1999; Herrero-Vanrell *et al.*, 2000; Moreira *et al.*, 1991; Bernatchez *et al.*, 1993; Gandolfi *et al.*, 1992 1997.
Nasal	Bioadhesion resulting in increased bioavailability	Xylometazoline, vasopressin, gentamycin	Morimoto *et al.*, 1991; Lim *et al.*, 2002.
Pulmonary	Absorption enhancer and dissolution rate modification	Insulin	Morimoto *et al.*, 2001; Surendrakumar *et al.*, 2003.
Parenteral	Drug carrier and facilitator of liposomal entrapment	Taxol, superoxide dismutase, human recombinant insulin-like growth factor, doxorubicin	Drobnik, 1991; Sakurai *et al.*, 1997; Luo and Prestwich, 1999; Luo *et al.*, 2000; Prisell *et al.*, 1992; Yerushalmi *et al.*, 1994; Yerushalmi & Margalit, 1998; Peer & Margalit, 2000; Eliaz & Szoka, 2001; Peer *et al.*, 2003.
Implant	Dissolution rate modification	Insulin	Surini *et al.*, 2003; Takayama *et al.*, 1990.
Gene	Dissolution rate modification and protection	Plasmid DNA/ monoclonal antibodies	Yun *et al.*, 2004; Kim *et al.*, 2003.

Open in a separate window
Cosmetic uses of hyaluronic acid

HA has been extensively utilized in cosmetic products because of its viscoelastic properties and excellent biocompatibility. Application of HA containing cosmetic products to the skin is reported to moisturize and restore elasticity, thereby achieving an antiwrinkle effect, albeit so far no rigorous scientific proof exists to substantiate this claim. HA-based cosmetic formulations or sunscreens may also be capable of protecting the skin against ultraviolet irradiation due to the free radical scavenging properties of HA (Manuskiatti & Maibach, 1996).

HA, either in a stabilized form or in combination with other polymers, is used as a component of commercial dermal fillers (e.g. Hylaform®, Restylane® and Dermalive®) in cosmetic surgery. It is reported that injection of such products into the dermis, can reduce facial lines and wrinkles in the long term with fewer side-effects and better tolerability compared with the use of collagen (Duranti et al., 1998; Bergeret-Galley et al., 2001; Leyden et al., 2003). The main side-effect may be an allergic reaction, possibly due to impurities present in HA (Schartz, 1997; Glogau, 2000).

Go to:
Biological function of hyaluronan

Naturally, hyaluronan has essential roles in body functions according to organ type in which it is distributed (Laurent et al., 1996).

Space filler

The specific functions of hyaluronan in joints are still essentially unknown. The simplest explanation for its presence would be that a flow of hyaluronan through the joint is needed to keep the joint cavity open and thereby allow extended movements of the joint. Hyaluronan is constantly secreted into the joint and removed by the synovium. The total amount of hyaluronan in the joint cavity is determined by these two processes. The half-life of the polysaccharide at steady-state is in the order of 0.5–1 day in rabbit and sheep (Brown *et al.,* 1991; Fraser *et al.,* 1993). The volume of the cavity is determined by the pressure conditions (hydrostatic and osmotic) in the cavity and its surroundings. Hyaluronan could, by its osmotic contributions and its formation of flow barriers in the limiting layers, be a regulator of the pressure and flow rate (McDonald & Leviek, 1995). It is interesting that in fetal development the formation of joint cavities is parallel with a local increase in hyaluronan (Edwards *et al.,* 1994).

Lubrication

Hyaluronan has been regarded as an ideal lubricant in the joints due to its shear-dependent viscosity (Ogston & Stanier, 1953) but its role in lubrication has been refuted by others (Radin *et al.,* 1970). However, there are now reasons to believe that the function of hyaluronan is to form a film between the cartilage surfaces. The load on the joints may press out water and low-molecular solutes from the hyaluronan layer into the cartilage matrix. As a result, the concentration of hyaluronan increases and a gel structure of micrometric thickness is formed which protects the cartilage surfaces from frictional damage (Hlavacek, 1993). This mechanism to form a protective layer is much less effective in arthritis when the synovial hyaluronan has both a lower concentration and a lower molecular weight than normal. Another change in the arthritic joint is the protein composition of the synovial fluid. Fraser *et al.* (1972) showed more than 40 years ago that addition of various serum proteins to hyaluronan substantially increased the viscosity and this has received a renewed interest in view of recently discovered hyaladherins (see above). TSG-6 and inter-α-trypsin inhibitor and other acute phase reactants such as haptoglobin are concentrated to arthritic synovial fluid (Hutadilok *et al.*, 1988). It is not known to what extent these are affecting the rheology and lubricating properties.

Scavenger functions

Hyaluronan has also been assigned scavenger functions in the joints. It has been known since the 1940s that hyaluronan is degraded by various oxidizing systems and ionizing irradiation and we know today that the common denominator is a chain cleavage induced by free radicals, essentially hydroxy radicals (Myint *et al.*, 1987). Through this reaction hyaluronan acts as a very efficient scavenger of free radicals. Whether this has any biological importance in protecting the joint against free radicals is unknown. The rapid turnover of hyaluronan in the joints has led to the suggestion that it also acts as a scavenger for cellular debris (Laurent *et al.*, 1995). Cellular material could be caught in the hyaluronan network and removed at the same rate as the polysaccharide (Stankovska *et al.*, 2007; Rapta, *et al.*, 2009).

Regulation of cellular activities

As discussed above, more recently proposed functions of hyaluronan are based on its specific interactions with hyaladherins. One interesting aspect is the fact that hyaluronan influences angiogenesis but the effect is different depending on its concentration and molecular weight (Sattar *et al.*, 1992). High molecular weight and high concentrations of the polymer inhibit the formation of capillaries, while oligosaccharides can induce angiogenesis. There are also reports of hyaluronan receptors on vascular endothelial cells by which hyaluronan could act on the cells (Edwards *et al.*, 1995). The avascularity of the joint cavity could be a result of hyaluronan inhibition of angiogenesis.

Another interaction of some interest in the joint is the binding of hyaluronan to cell surface proteins. Lymphocytes and other cells may find their way to joints through this interaction. Injection of high doses of hyaluronan intra-articularly could attract cells expressing these proteins. Cells can also change their expression of hyaluronan-binding proteins in states of disease, whereby hyaluronan may influence immunological reactions and cellular traffic in the path of physiological processes in cells (Edwards *et al.,* 1995). The observation often reported that intra-articular injections of hyaluronan alleviate pain in joint disease (Adams, 1993) may indicate a direct or indirect interaction with pain receptors.

Go to:
Hyaluronan and synovial fluid

In normal/healthy joint, the synovial fluid, which consists of an ultrafiltrate of blood plasma and glycoproteins contains HA macromolecules of molar mass ranging between 6–10 mega Daltons (Praest *et al.,* 1997). SF serves also as a lubricating and shock absorbing boundary layer between moving parts of synovial joints. SF reduces friction and wear and tear of the synovial joint playing thus a vital role in the lubrication and protection of the joint tissues from damage during motion (Oates *et al.,* 2002).

As SF of healthy humans exhibits no activity of hyaluronidase, it has been inferred that oxygen-derived free radicals are involved in a self-perpetuating process of HA catabolism within the joint (Grootveld *et al.,* 1991; Stankovska *et al.,* 2006; Rychly *et al.,* 2006). This radical-mediated process is considered to account for ca. twelve-hour half-life of native HA macromolecules in SF.

Acceleration of degradation of high-molecular-weight HA occurring under inflammation and/or oxidative stress is accompanied by impairment and loss of its viscoelastic properties (Parsons *et al.,* 2002; Soltes *et al.,* 2005; Stankovska *et al.,* 2005; Lath *et al.,* 2005; Hrabarova *et al.,* 2007; Valachova & Soltes, 2010; Valachova *et al.,* 2013a). Low-molecular weight HA was found to exert different biological activities compared to the native high-molecular-weight biopolymer. HA chains of 25–50 disaccharide units are inflammatory, immune-stimulatory, and highly angiogenic. HA fragments of this size appear to function as endogenous danger signals, reflecting tissues under stress (Noble, 2002; West *et al.,* 1985; Soltes *et al.,* 2007; Stern *et al.,* 2007; Soltes & Kogan, 2009). **Figure 5** describes the fragmentation mechanism of HA under free radical stress.

- Initiation phase: the intact hyaluronan macromolecule entering the reaction with the HO· radical formed via the Fenton-like reaction:
- $Cu_+ + H_2O_2 \rightarrow Cu_{2+} + HO· + OH_-$
- H_2O_2 has its origin due to the oxidative action of the Weissberger system (see **Figure 6**)

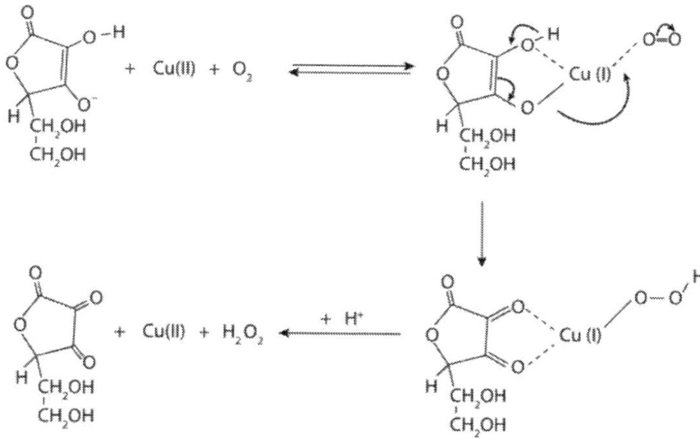

Figure 6

Scheme. Generation of H_2O_2 by Weissberger's system from ascorbate and Cu(II) ions under aerobic conditions (Valachova *et al.,* 2011)

- Formation of an alkyl radical (C-centered hyaluronan

macroradical) initiated by the HO· radical attack.

- Propagation phase: formation of a peroxy-type C-macroradical of hyaluronan in a process of oxygenation after entrapping a molecule of O_2.
- Formation of a hyaluronan-derived hydroperoxide via the reaction with another hyaluronan macromolecule.
- Formation of highly unstable alkoxy-type C-macroradical of hyaluronan on undergoing a redox reaction with a transition metal ion in a reduced state.
- Termination phase: quick formation of alkoxy-type C-fragments and the fragments with a terminal C=O group due to the glycosidic bond scission of hyaluronan. Alkoxy-type C fragments may continue the propagation phase of the free-radical hyaluronan degradation reaction. Both fragments are represented by reduced molar masses (Kogan, 2011; Rychly *et al.,* 2006; Hrabarova *et al.,* 2012; Surovcikova *et al.,* 2012; Valachova *et al.,* 2013b; Banasova *et al.,* 2012).

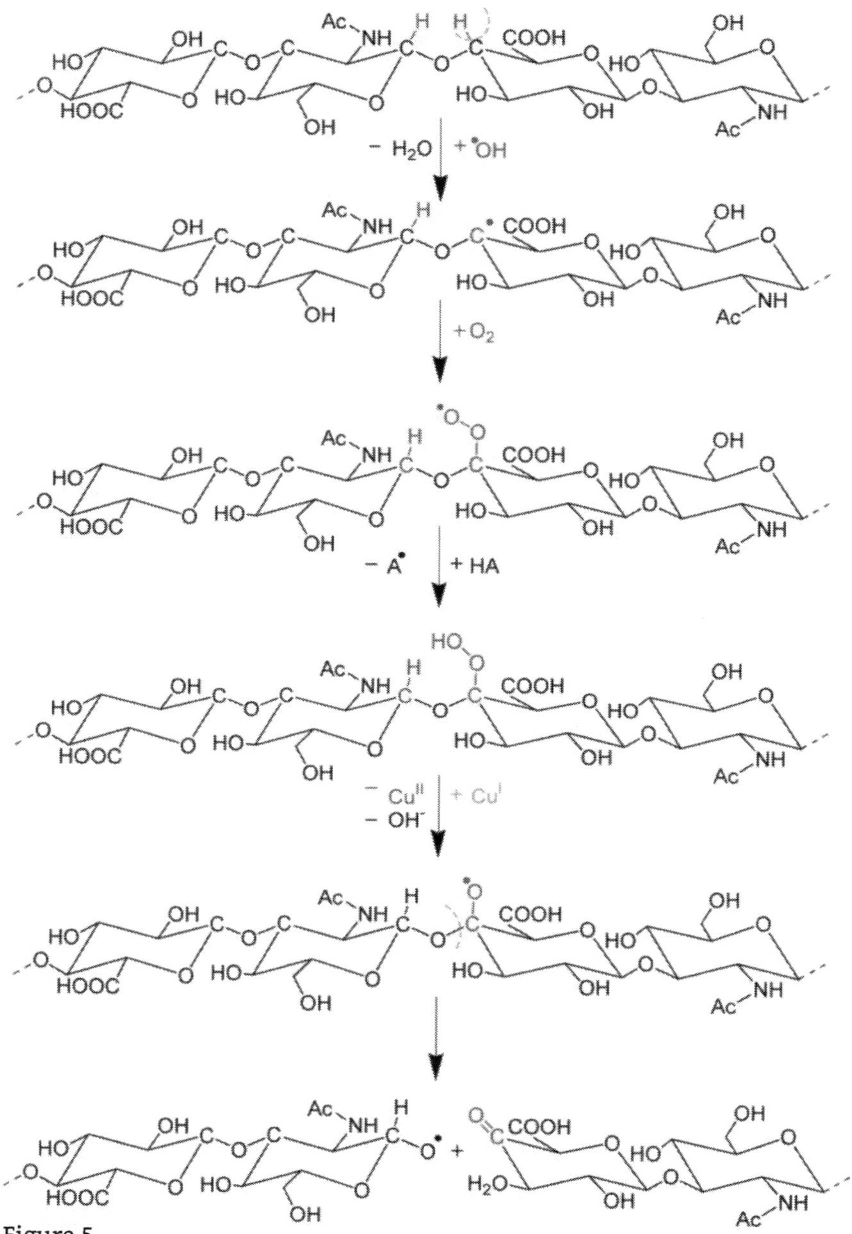

Figure 5

Schematic degradation of HA under free radical stress (Hrabarova *et al.*, 2012).

Several thiol compounds have attracted much attention from pharmacologists because of their reactivity toward endobiotics such as hydroxyl radical-derived species. Thiols play an important role as biological reductants (antioxidants) preserving the redox status of cells and protecting tissues against damage caused by the elevated reactive oxygen/nitrogen species (ROS/RNS) levels, by which oxidative stress might be indicated.

Soltes and his coworkers examined the effect of several thiol compounds on inhibition of the degradation kinetics of a high-molecular-weight HA *In vitro*. High molecular weight hyaluronan samples were exposed to free-radical chain degradation reactions induced by ascorbate in the presence of Cu(II) ions, the so called Weissberger's oxidative system. The concentrations of both reactants [ascorbate, Cu(II)] were comparable to those that may occur during an early stage of the acute phase of joint inflammation (see **Figure 6**) (Banasova *et al.*, 2011; Valachova *et al.*, 2011; Soltes *et al.*, 2006a; Soltes *et al.*, 2006b; Stankovska *et al.*, 2004; Soltes *et al.*, 2006c; Soltes *et al.*, 2007; Valachova *et al.*, 2008; 2009; 2010; 2011; 2013; Hrabarova *et al.*, 2009, 2011; Rapta *et al.*, 2009; 2010; Surovcikova-Machova *et al.*, 2012; Banasova *et al.*, 2011; Drafi *et al.*, 2010; Fisher & Naughton, 2005).

Figure 7 illustrates the dynamic viscosity of hyaluronan solution in the presence and absence of bucillamine, d-penicillamine and l-cysteine as inhibitors for free radical degradation of HA. The study showed that bucillamine to be both a preventive and chain-breaking antioxidant. On the other hand, d-penicillamine and l-cysteine dose dependently act as scavenger of ·OH radicals within the first 60 min. Then, however, the inhibition activity is lost and degradation of hyaluronan takes place (Valachova *et al.*, 2011; Valachova *et al.*, 2009; 2010; Hrabarova *et al.*, 2009).

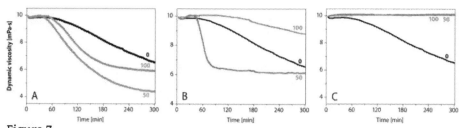

Figure 7

Effect of **A)** l-penicillamine, **B)** l-cysteine and **C)** bucillamine with different concentrations (50, 100 µM) on HA degradation induced by the oxidative system containing 1.0 µM CuCl₂ + 100 µM ascorbic acid (Valachova *et al.*, 2011).

l-Glutathione (GSH; l-γ-glutamyl-l-cysteinyl-glycine; a ubiquitous endogenous thiol, maintains the intracellular reduction-oxidation (redox) balance and regulates signaling pathways during oxidative stress/conditions. GSH is mainly cytosolic in the concentration range of ca. 1–10 mM; however, in the plasma as well as in SF, the range is only 1–3 µM (Haddad & Harb, 2005). This unique thiol plays a crucial role in antioxidant defense, nutrient metabolism, and in regulation of pathways essential for the whole body homeostasis. Depletion of GSH results in an increased vulnerability of the cells to oxidative stress (Hultberg & Hultberg, 2006).

It was found that l-glutathione exhibited the most significant protective and chain-breaking antioxidative effect against hyaluronan degradation. Thiol antioxidative activity, in general, can be influenced by many factors such as various molecule geometry, type of functional groups, radical attack accessibility, redox potential, thiol concentration and pK$_a$, pH, ionic strength of solution, as well as different ability to interact with transition metals (Hrabarova *et al.*, 2012).

Figure 8 shows the dynamic viscosity versus time profiles of HA solution stressed to degradation with Weissberger's oxidative system. As evident, addition of different concentrations of GSH resulted in a marked protection of the HA macromolecules against degradation. The greater the GSH concentration used, the longer was the observed stationary interval in the sample viscosity values. At the lowest GSH concentration used, *i.e.* 1.0 μM (**Figure 8**), the time-dependent course of the HA degradation was more rapid than that of the reference experiment with the zero thiol concentration. Thus, one could classify GSH traces as functioning as a pro-oxidant.

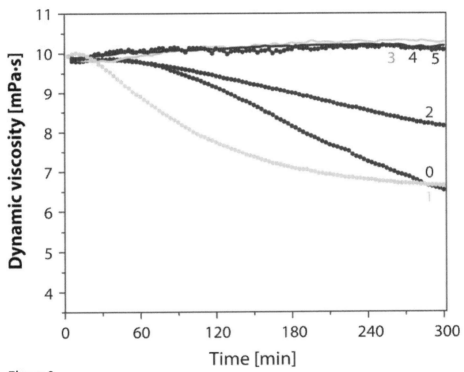

Figure 8
Comparison of the effect of l-glutathione on HA degradation induced by the system containing 1.0 μM CuCl₂ plus 100 μM l-ascorbic acid. Concentration of l-glutathione in μM: 1–1.0; 2–10; 3, 4, 5–50, 100, and 200. Concentration of reference experiment: 0–nil thiol concentration (Hrabarova *et al.*, 2009; Valachova *et al.*, 2010a).

The effectiveness of antioxidant activity of 1,4-dithioerythritol expressed as the radical scavenging capacity was studied by a rotational viscometry method (Hrabarova *et al.*, 2010). 1,4-dithioerythritol, widely accepted and used as an effective antioxidant in the field of enzyme and protein oxidation, is a new potential antioxidant standard exhibiting very good solubility in a variety of solvents. **Figure 9** describes the effect of 1,4-dithioerythritol on degradation of HA solution under free radical stress (Hrabarova *et al.*, 2010).

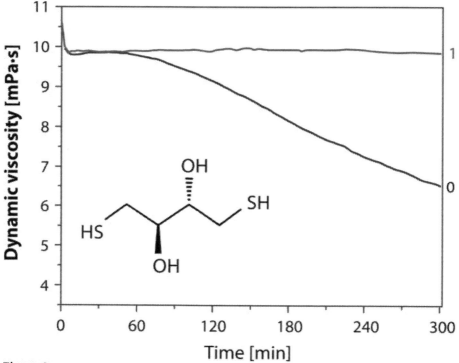

Figure 9

Effect of 1,4-dithioerythritol (1) on HA degradation induced by Weissberger's oxidative system (0) (Hrabarova *et al.*, 2010).

N-Acetyl-l-cysteine (NAC), another significant precursor of the GSH biosynthesis, has broadly been used as effective antioxidant in a form of nutritional supplement (Soloveva *et al.*, 2007; Thibodeau *et al.*, 2001). At low concentrations, it is a powerful protector of α_1-antiproteinase against the enzyme inactivation by HOCl. NAC reacts with HO· radicals and slowly with H_2O_2; however, no reaction of this endobiotic with superoxide anion radical was detected (Aruoma *et al.*, 1989).

Investigation of the antioxidative effect of *N*-Acetyl-l-cysteine. Unlike l-glutathione, *N*-acetyl-l-cysteine was found to have preferential tendency to reduce Cu(II) ions to Cu(I), forming *N*-acetyl-l-cysteinyl radical that may subsequently react with molecular O_2 to give O_2 – (Soloveva *et al.*, 2007; Thibodeau *et al.*, 2001). Contrary to l-cysteine, NAC (25 and 50 μM), when added at the beginning of the reaction, exhibited a clear antioxidative effect within ca. 60 and 80 min, respectively (**Figure 10A**). Subsequently, NAC exerted a modest pro-oxidative effect, more profound at 25-μM than at 100-μM concentration (**Figure 10A**). Application of NAC 1 h after the onset of the reaction (**Figure 10B**) revealed its partial inhibitory effect against formation of the peroxy-type radicals, independently from the concentration applied (Hrabarova *et al.*, 2012).

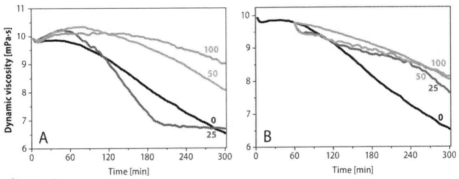

Figure 10

Evaluation of antioxidative effects of *N*-acetyl-l-cysteine against high-molar-mass hyaluronan degradation *in vitro* induced by Weissberger's oxidative system. Reference sample (black): 1 M Cu(II) ions plus 100 μM ascorbic acid; nil thiol concentration. *N*-Acetyl-l-cysteine addition at the onset of the reaction (A) and after 1 h (B) (25, 50,100 μM). (Hrabarova *et al.*, 2012).

An endogenous amine, cysteamine (CAM) is a cystine-depleting compound with antioxidative and anti-inflammatory properties; it is used for treatment of cystinosis – a metabolic disorder caused by deficiency of the lysosomal cystine carrier. CAM is widely distributed in organisms and considered to be a key regulator of essential metabolic pathways (Kessler *et al.*, 2008).

Investigation of the antioxidative effect of cysteamine. Cysteamine (100 μM), when added before the onset of the reaction, exhibited an antioxidative effect very similar to that of GSH (**Figure 8A** and **Figure 11A**). Moreover, the same may be concluded when applied 1 h after the onset of the reaction (**Figure 11B**) at the two concentrations (50 and 100 μM), suggesting that CAM may be an excellent scavenger of peroxy radicals generated during the peroxidative degradation of HA (Hrabarova *et al.*, 2012).

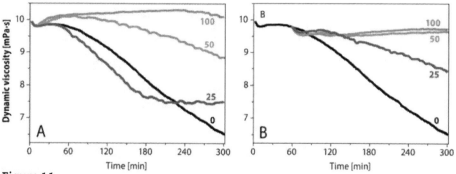

Figure 11

Evaluation of antioxidative effects of cysteamine against high-molar-mass hyaluronan degradation *in vitro* induced by Weissberger's oxidative system. Reference sample (black): 1 mM CuII ions plus 100μM ascorbic acid; nil thiol concentration. Cysteamine addition at the onset of the reaction (a) and after 1 h (b) (25, 50,100 μM). (Hrabarova *et al.*, 2012).

Involvement of transposable elements in neurogenesis

R.N. Mustafin and E.K. Khusnutdinova
Author information Article notes Copyright and License information PMC Disclaimer

Go to:

Abstract

The article is about the role of transposons in the regulation of functioning of neuronal stem cells and mature neurons of the human brain. Starting from the first division of the zygote, embryonic development is governed by regular activations of transposable elements, which are necessary for the sequential regulation of the expression of genes specific for each cell type. These processes include differentiation of neuronal stem cells, which requires the finest tuning of expression of neuron genes in various regions of the brain. Therefore, in the hippocampus, the center of human neurogenesis, the highest transposon activity has been identified, which causes somatic mosaicism of cells during the formation of specific brain structures. Similar data were obtained in studies on experimental animals. Mobile genetic elements are the most important sources of long non-coding RNAs that are coexpressed with important brain protein-coding genes. Significant activity of long non-coding RNA was detected in the hippocampus, which confirms the role of transposons in the regulation of brain function. MicroRNAs, many of which arise from transposon transcripts, also play an important role in regulating the differentiation of neuronal stem cells. Therefore, transposons, through their own processed transcripts, take an active part in the epigenetic regulation of differentiation of neurons. The global regulatory role of transposons in the human brain is due to the emergence of protein-coding genes in evolution by their exonization, duplication and domestication. These genes are involved in an epigenetic regulatory network with the participation of transposons, since they contain nucleotide sequences complementary to miRNA and long non-coding RNA formed from transposons. In the memory formation, the role of the exchange of virus-like mRNA with the help of the Arc protein of endogenous retroviruses HERV between neurons has been revealed. A possible mechanism for the implementation of this mechanism may be reverse transcription of mRNA and site-specific insertion into the genome with a regulatory effect on the genes involved in the memory.

Keywords: brain, differentiation, noncoding RNA, retroelements, neuronal stem cells, transposable elements

Go to:

Introduction

Transposable elements (TE) make up 69 % of the human genome (de Koning et al., 2011). In the course of evolution, many protein-coding genes (Joly-Lopez, Bureau, 2018), regulatory nucleotide sequences (Ito et al., 2017; Schrader, Schmitz, 2018), and telomeres (Kopera et al., 2011), non-coding RNAs (ncRNAs), including microRNAs (Piriyapongsa et al., 2007; Yuan et al., 2010, 2011; Qin et al., 2015) and long human ncRNAs (Johnson, Guigo, 2014) originating from TE. Over millions of years of evolution, cells have developed various defense systems against TE insertion into their genomes, including DNA methylation, heterochromatin formation, and RNA interference (RNAi). These epigenetic mechanisms have made a significant contribution to the regulation of specific gene expression and cell differentiation (Habibi et al., 2015).

Transposable elements are divided into two main classes, in accordance with the mechanisms of their transposition. DNA-TEs are transposed by "cut and paste" or "rolling circle". Retroelements (REs) are integrated into new genome sites using "copy and paste". REs are classified into those containing long terminal repeats (LTR REs) (Fig. 1) and those not containing them (non-LTR REs) (Fig. 2). The latter are divided into autonomous (LINE, long interspersed nuclear elements) and non-autonomous (SINE, short interspersed nuclear elements) and SVA (SINE-VNTR-Alu) (Fig. 3) (Klein, O'Neill, 2018).

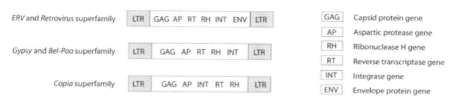

Fig. 1.
Scheme of the structure of the genes of LTR-containing retroelements.

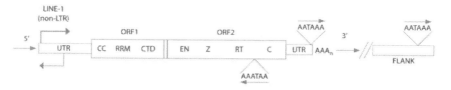

Fig. 2.
Scheme of the structure of the gene of non-LTR retroelements (LINE-1).
UTR – untranslated region; ORF – open reading frame; CC – coiled-coiled; RRM – RNA recognition motif; CTD – C-terminal domain; EN – endonuclease; Z – Z-domain; RT – reverse transcriptase; C – cysteine-rich domain.

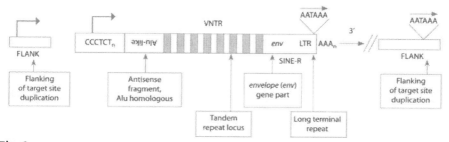

Fig. 3.
Scheme of the structure of SVA elements.

The human genome contains more than 500,000 copies of LINE1 (L1), which make up 17 % of all nucleotide sequences. Among them, only about 100 L1 are active, since they contain the full length of 6000 bp. Among non-autonomous REs, the human genome contains more than 2700 copies of SVA (Hancks, Kazazian, 2012). One of the important factors for the development of the human brain is considered the waves of L1 retrotranspositions, as well as the birth of new TEs, such as SINE, Alu and SVA in the evolution of primates (Linker et al., 2017).

Human endogenous retroviruses (HERV) belong to LTRRE. They occupy about 8 % of the entire genome and serve as sources of a huge number (794,972) of binding sites with specific transcription factors (TFs), the activation of which plays a role in embryogenesis. For example, in the mesoderm, LTRs interact with SOX17, FOXA1, GATA4; in pluripotent cells, with SOX2, NANOG, POU5F1; in hematopoietic cells, with TAL1, GATA1, PU1 (Ito et al., 2017). Mammalian-wide interspersed repeats (MIRs), which belong to the ancient SINE family descended from tRNA, are also associated with tissuespecific gene expression (Jjingo et al., 2014).

Transposable elements are characterized by nonrandom activation, depending on the tissue and stage of development. High-throughput profiling of integration sites by nextgeneration sequencing, combined with large-scale genomic data mining and cellular or biochemical approaches, has revealed that the insertions are usually non-random (Sultana et al., 2017). Programmed activation of TE in individual cells during neurogenesis leads to a change in the expression of certain genes necessary for differentiation into specific types of neurons for the formation and functioning of brain structures (Coufal et al., 2009; Bailie et al., 2011; Thomas, Muotri, 2012; Richardson et al., 2014; Evrony et al., 2015; Upton et al., 2015; Muotri, 2016; Suarez et al., 2018). In accordance with this, somatic mosaicism of neurons detected by insertions of TEs (Richardson et al., 2014; Upton et al., 2015; Bachiller et al., 2017; Paquola et al., 2017; Rohrback et al., 2018; Suarez et al.,

2018) can reflect the programmed regulatory pattern of the genome necessary for the maturation of specific structures of the central nervous system (Paquola et al., 2017; Rohrback et al., 2018). Somatic mosaicism means the presence, in the same organism, of cells with different genomes as a result of de novo DNA changes. These structural variations may be due to CNV, insertions of REs, deletions under the influence of TEs, and SNV (Paquola et al., 2017). This means that in different cells of one organism, not only the genotype, but also the whole genome changes. This is due to the occurrence of mutations in exons of protein-coding genes, intergenic regulatory regions and introns, which is accompanied by a specific expression of certain genes specific for each cell type.

Go to:

The role of transposable elements in neuronal differentiation

The human brain contains an average of 86.1 billion neurons. Moreover, each of the neurons forms from 5,000 to 20,000 synaptic connections, creating a complex network with a variety of cell types and subtypes. The number of subtypes of neurons is so large that it does not lend itself to modern methods for their description. There must be mechanisms to ensure such a diversity of neurons with their specific temporal and spatial features of functioning (Thomas, Muotri, 2012). The sources of these mechanisms can be TEs, combinations of movements of which can become sources of countless variety. An example of this is the molecular mechanism for generating antibodies by the mammalian immune system (V(D)J recombination), derived from TEs (Lapp, Hunter, 2016). TEs played a role in the development of the central nervous system. In evolution, they turned out to be sources of the formation of regulatory structures and genes involved in the formation of the brain. Non-autonomous TEs MER130 were preserved in the genomes during evolution due to their location near the neocortex genes as a necessary link for their regulation. The experiments showed the activation of MER130 in mouse embryos on the fourteenth day of development as gene enhancers for the development of the neocortex (Notwell et al., 2015). Among 11 sushi-ichi-specific placental animal genes derived from REs, the SIRH11/ZCCHC16 gene encoding zinc finger CCHC protein contributed to the evolution of the brain. This domesticated gene is involved in the development of cognitive functions of placental animals (Irie et al., 2016).

In 2009, in neuronal stem cells isolated from the brain of a human embryo, L1s retrotranspositions were detected, as well as an increase (in comparison with the liver and heart of the same individual) in the number of copies of endogenous L1s in the adult hippocampus (Coufal et al., 2009). In addition to L1 (7743 insertions), a large number of somatic transpositions Alu (13,692 insertions) and SVA (1350 insertions) were found in the hippocampus of adults (Bailie et al., 2011). These de novo integrations can affect the expression of certain genes, creating unique transcriptomes of individual neurons (Muotri, 2016). This may be due to the genome-programmed TE ability for their regular site-specific insertions (Sultana et al., 2017). In 2009, of 19 retrotranspositions, 16 were found at a distance of less than 100 kilobases from genes expressed in neurons (Coufal et al., 2009). In 2015, in a study of the somatic mosaicism of the human hippocampus K.R. Upton et al. revealed, out of 20 identified L1 transpositions, 2 functionally significant insertions into the introns of the ZFAND3 and USP33 genes functioning in the brain (Upton et al., 2015). A.A. Kurnosov et al., when studying human brain samples, showed that out of 3100 transpositions of L1 in neurons of the dentate gyrus of the hippocampus, 50.26 % of insertions are located in the genes, and out of 2984 Alu, 49.1 % (Kurnosov et al., 2015). In 2016, J.A. Erwin et al. revealed that in the brain of healthy people 44–63 % of neurons undergo somatic mosaicism at the loci of genes that are important for the functioning of the nervous system. For example, a high insertion frequency of L1-RE is shown for the DLG2 gene, which affects cognitive flexibility, attention, and learning. Mutations in DLG2 are associated with the development of schizophrenia (Erwin et al., 2016).

Somatic retrotranspositions, unlike germinal ones, cannot be inherited by future generations. However, the programmed ability for specific insertions, depending on the composition and location of TEs in the genome, can be inherited. An explanation of the ability of TEs to be inserted in a site-specific manner in the region of genes expressed in the brain may be the evolutionary relationship of protein-coding genes and their regulatory sequences with TEs (Gianfrancesco et al., 2017; Ito et al., 2017; Joly-Lopez, Bureau, 2018). The insertions specific for humans and chimpanzees were revealed near the promoters of the tachycin receptor genes TACR3, cation channels TRPV1 and TRPV3, oxytocin OXT. These genes are associated with the functioning of neuropeptides. Analysis of the genomes of various mammals showed that the neural enhancer nPE2, which regulates the expression of the POMC gene in the hypothalamus, evolved from SINE in evolution (Gianfrancesco et al., 2017).

Transpositions and expression of TEs can vary depending on the area of the brain and change under environmental influences, as they can perform a number of adaptive functions (Lapp, Hunter, 2016). More active are L1, which retained the ability to transpose, causing somatic mosaicism (Suarez et al., 2018). In 2005, A.R. Muotri et al. suggested that L1 using somatic transpositions can actively create mosaicism of neuron genomes (Muotri et al., 2005). In the brain, somatic mosaicism plays an important role in the regulation of cognition and behavior. The consequences of somatic mosaicism encompass vast changes – from a variant at a single locus, to genes in neuronal networks (Paquola et al., 2017; Rohrback et al., 2018). Moreover, the features of somatic mosaicism differ between neurons of various regions of the brain. For example, in the cerebral cortex, only 0.6 insertions of L1-RE are observed, while in the hippocampus, from 80 to 800 inserts per neuron (Lapp, Hunter, 2016). Somatic mosaicism due to retrotranspositions is a source of phenotypic diversity between neurons during development. In the brain of an adult under the influence of various environmental factors, L1 expression can affect the functioning of neurons during the formation of long-term memory (Bachiller et al., 2017).

The hippocampus is the center of human neurogenesis, where many insertions affect transcriptional expression, creating unique transcriptomes in neurons. In addition, transcriptional activation of L1 is similar to that for the NeuroD1 gene. This may indicate the effect of L1 expression on neurogenesis, since stimulation of Wnt3a in neuronal stem cells increases L1 expression 10-fold along the beta-catenin pathway, similarly activating transcription of the NeuroD1 gene. This gene encodes the transcription factor that activates the genes involved in neurogenesis. The NeuroD1 promoter region contains a Sox/ LEF site similar to the 5′UTR of the L1 element, and the pattern of time expression of the NeuroD1 and L1 genes during differentiation of neurons is similar (Thomas, Muotri, 2012).

Genetic variations between neurons due to L1 retrotranspositions may be associated with specific enrichment of neuronal stem cell enhancers. It was shown that specific enhancers for certain types of neurons (determined using FANTOM5) correspond to the coordinates in the genome for insertions L1, which are within 100 bp from the enhancer. These patterns have not been identified for astrocytes and hepatocytes (Upton et al., 2015). When studying the features of L1 retrotranspositions in more than 30 regions of the brain, a lot of L1 insertion-specific cell lines were found (Evrony et al., 2015). In experiments on mice, specific L1 expression was also shown depending on the area of the brain and the age of the animal (Cappucci et al., 2018).

In addition to L1 elements, LTR-REs are also involved in the regulation of neurogenesis. For example, in mice, the region where the full-length ERVmch8 on chromosome 8 was located was comparatively less methylated in the cerebellum, due to its specific expression depending on the stage of development (Lee et al., 2011). In accordance with these data, it can be assumed that the features of TEs activation observed in neuronal stem cells can naturally alter the expression of specific genes necessary for differentiation of neurons during the formation of specific brain structures. The reason for the activation of TEs in the neuronal stem cells of the hippocampus and the reason for their importance in memory consolidation may be the sensitivity of TEs to stressful environmental influences (Mustafin, Khusnutdinova, 2019). These mechanisms are a particular reflection of the general pattern of epigenetic control of the development of the whole organism, starting from the first division of the zygote, under the regulatory influence of TEs (Mustafin, Khusnutdinova, 2018). To understand the role of TEs in these processes, it is necessary to consider their participation in embryogenesis.

Go to:

The role of transposable elements in embryogenesis

To initiate the development of the body after fertilization, gametes are reprogrammed to totipotency. During this reprogramming, TEs activation is observed. Previously, this phenomenon was believed to be a side effect of extensive chromatin remodeling at the basis of epigenetic reprogramming of gametes. However, a targeted epigenomic approach has been performed to determine whether TEs directly affect chromatin organization and body development. It was found that silencing of L1 elements reduces the availability of chromatin, and prolonged activation of L1 prevents its gradual compaction, which occurs naturally during development. That is, L1 activation is an integral part of the development program (Jachowicz et al., 2017). In experiments on mice, the role of LTR-REs as a necessary control element for early embryogenesis was proved (Wang et al., 2016).

For the cis-regulatory activity of the LTR retroelements ERVK, MERVL and GLN, a complex of RNA and proteins is required, formed using the long ncRNA LincGET. Artificial silencing of LincGET expression in the embryo at the bicellular stage leads to a complete halt to further development due to disruption of cis-regulation of the genes necessary for proliferation under the influence of LTR-REs driven by LincGET (Wang et al., 2016). It has also been shown that HERVs are activated in all types of human cells with characteristic features for certain tissues and organs (Seifarth et al., 2005). In the study of the association of 112 TE families in 24 human tissues, tissue-specific enrichment of active regions of LTR-REs was noted, which indicates the involvement of LTE-REs in the regulation of gene expression for differentiation of cells depending on their functional purpose in ontogenesis. This is due to the presence, in the TEs sequences, of transcription factors binding sites (TFBSs) that regulate the development of the corresponding tissue. TE enrichment characteristic of certain cells in intron enhancers correlates with tissue-specific variations in the expression of nearby genes (Trizzino et al., 2018).

The genetic program in the 2-cell stage of embryogenesis in mice and humans is largely controlled by transcription factors of the DUX family, which are key inducers of zygote genome activation in placental mammals (De Laco et al., 2017). L1 transcripts in embryos are necessary for Dux silencing, rRNA synthesis and exit from the 2-cell stage. M. Percharde et al. in their article showed that L1 expression is required for preimplantation development (Percharde et al., 2018). In embryonic cells, L1 transcripts act as a nuclear RNA scaffold that recruits Nucleolin and Kap1/Trim28 factors for Dux repression. In parallel, L1 products mediate the binding of Nucleolin and Kap1 to rDNA, contributing to the synthesis of rRNA and self-renewal of embryonic stem cells (Percharde et al., 2018). The role of L1 in the repression of the transcriptional program of a 2-cell embryo indicates their participation in the development-specific regulation of gene expression necessary for cell differentiation and body development (Jachowicz et al., 2017). It can be assumed that the activity of REs in neuronal stem cells indicates their use as switches of transcription programs in the specific functionalization of neurons. That is, TEs are involved in the management of both the differentiation of embryonic cells and postnatal stem cells. Regulation is carried out by implementing information encoded in the features of the composition and distribution of TEs in the genome, through the sequential activation of strictly defined TEs in each new cell, specific for the tissue and stage of development. The greatest role is played by this species-specific "coding" in the brain, where neurons are distinguished by higher activity of REs. This is reflected in the structural and functional complexity of the brain compared to other organs. The use of TEs as sources of ncRNAs plays an important role in these processes.

Go to:

The relationship of transposable elements with non-coding RNAs in the brain

According to recent data, from 75 to 85 % of the human genome is transcribed into primary transcripts, while only 1.2 % of the genome is translated into proteins. Most transcripts are registered as ncRNAs that are involved in the regulation of the genome (Djebali et al., 2012). In humans, 13,000 genes of long ncRNAs have been identified, for the occurrence of which HERVs are responsible by insertion of promoters. HERV-stimulated long ncRNAs are characterized by specific transcription in different types of pluripotent cells, which is consistent with the over-expression of these HERVs in human embryonic stem cells (Johnson, Guigo, 2014). Transcription of most long ncRNAs is associated with the expression of protein coding genes according to the type of neurons and a specific region of the brain. For example, according to Allen Brain Atlas in situ hybridization data, out of 1328 known long mouse ncRNAs, 849 are expressed in their brain and are associated with cell types and subcellular structures. The biological significance of these ncRNAs in the functioning of neurons and their relationship with protein-coding genes has been shown (Mercer et al., 2008).

Long ncRNAs expressed in the brain, such as Miat, Rmst, Gm17566, Gm14207, Gm16758, 2610307P16Rik, C230034O21Rik, 9930014A18Rik, share a similar expression model with neurogenesis genes and overlap these genes, which proves the role of long ncRNAs in neurogenesis (Aprea et al., 2013). These data are consistent with the role of TEs in neurogenesis (Coufal et al., 2009; Kurnosov et al., 2015; Erwin et al., 2016; Muotri, 2016) and regulation of brain function (Thomas, Muotri, 2012; Upton et al., 2015; Rohrback et al., 2018). This is because TEs are the main sources of the emergence and evolution of long ncRNAs, forming their functional domains and making up more than 2/3 of their mature transcripts in humans (Kapusta, Feschotte, 2014). REs can serve as genes for long ncRNAs (Lu et al., 2014). L1s have a function similar to lncRNA in regulating the expression of genes necessary for self-renewal of stem cells and for preimplantation development (Honson, Macfarlan, 2018).

In a number of studies, the role of miRNAs in controlling the differentiation of neurons, switching expression profiles of genes important for cell function in time and space has been proved (Stappert et al., 2015). About 40 % of all known human miRNAs are expressed in the human brain. The specific expression of many of them differs in different types of cells and is important in the regulation of differentiation, which is necessary for a huge variety of phenotypes of neurons in the brain (Smirnova et al., 2005). The accumulation of certain miRNAs in various structures of neurons (axons, dendrites, synapses) was revealed. For example, in experiments in mice, the role of miR-134 in the regulation of specific mRNAs of the LIMK1 gene for the growth of dendritic spins was shown, and the accumulation of miR-99a, 124a1-3, 125b1, 125b2, 134, 339 was noted in synaptosomes (Lugli et al., 2008). The formation of neurites is promoted by miR-21 (the target is the mRNA of the SPRY2 gene), miR-431 is involved in the regeneration of axons (the target is the Kremen-1 gene), differentiation of neurons occurs under the influence of miR- 34a (the targets are Tap73, synaptotagmin-1, syntaxin-1A) and miR-137 (targets are the Mib1, Ezh2 genes). Enhanced expression of miR-9 promotes branching and reduced axon growth by repressing microtubule-associated Map1b protein. Axon growth depends on the effect of miR-431, as well as miR-17-92, which interacts with PTEN (phosphate tensin homolog) in neurons of the cerebral cortex of the embryo. The regulatory role of differential expression of miR-221 and miR-222 in neurogenesis has also been proven (Nampoothiri, Rajanikant, 2017).

In 2007, J. Piriyapongsa et al. found that in humans TEs can be sources of microRNAs (Piriyapongsa et al., 2007), which was confirmed by other researchers (Yuan et al., 2010, 2011; Qin et al., 2015). The key role of TEs in the formation of microRNAs and long ncRNAs (Johnson, Guigo, 2014; Ka-pusta, Feschotte, 2014) indicates that the maximum activity of TEs at the center of human neurogenesis (Kurnosov et al., 2015) as a natural phenomenon is necessary for epigenetic control of differentiation of neuronal stem cells. Another mechanism of TE participation in the regulation of gene expression necessary for the specific work of neurons is the cisand trans-effects of TEs (Garcia-Perez et al., 2016). This confirms the nonrandom activations of TEs as sources of heterogeneous subpopulations of neurons (Fig. 4) (Faulkner, 2011).

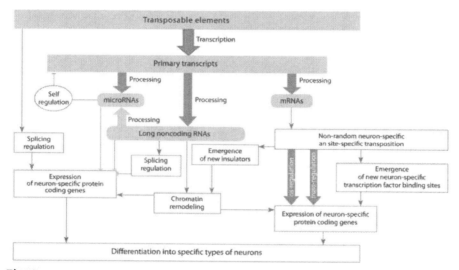

Fig. 4.
Scheme of TE involvement in neurogenesis.

Go to:

The role of retroelements in interactions between neurons

For the development and functioning of the brain, intercellular interactions are necessary, the study of the regulation mechanisms of which is promising for therapeutic targeted exposure to the work of the brain. For this, it is important to identify drivers for gene expression and post-transcriptional epigenetic regulation of the structural components of neurons. Based on the analysis of the accumulated data on the role of TEs in controlling the functioning of the genome in embryonic development (Garcia-Perez et al., 2007; Van den Hurk et al., 2007; Macia et al., 2011; Kurnosov et al., 2015; Percharde et al., 2018) and the physiological functioning of the human brain (Coufal et al., 2009; Bailie et al., 2011; Thomas, Muotri, 2012; Richardson et al., 2014; Evrony et al., 2015; Upton et al., 2015; Muotri, 2016; Suarez et al., 2018), it was concluded that TEs are regulators of epigenetic control for gene function in ontogenesis (Mustafin, Khusnutdinova, 2017, 2018). Despite the lack of mitotic activity of mature neurons, the specific expression of TEs in them is important in controlling both interneuronal interactions and the structural and functional characteristics of neurons (Bailie et al., 2011; Richardson et al., 2014; Erwin et al., 2016). These properties may be due to processing from transcripts of transposons of specific long ncRNAs (Lu et al., 2014; Honson, Macfarlan, 2018) and microRNAs (Piriyapongsa et al., 2007; Yuan et al., 2010, 2011; Qin et al., 2015). Indeed, in experiments on laboratory animals, the enrichment of specific miRNAs in certain structures and regions of neurons was revealed. For example, an abundance of miR-15b, miR-16, miR-204, miR-221 was found in the distal axons compared to neuron bodies (Natera-Naranjo et al., 2010). Enrichment of specific miRNAs in synapses was detected. This suggests a local post-transcriptional regulation of the expression of neuron-specific genes (Lugli et al., 2008). The role of miRNAs in intercellular interactions in the brain was shown, as well as the value of the electrical activity of neurons for the secretion of miR-124 and miR-9, which can penetrate microglia and change the phenotype of its cells (Veremeyko et al., 2019).

Transposable elements regulate brain function through expression into specific microRNAs that regulate gene expression in neurons and in intercellular interactions in the brain. The role of ERV in transferring information between neurons for memory consolidation has also been identified. In the human genome, the full-length HERV-K (about 10,000 bp) consists of the remains of ancient retroviruses and includes LTR-flanked regions, including three retroviral ORFs: pol-pro (encodes protease, RT and integrase enzymes), env (encodes horizontal transfer proteins) and gag (encodes structural proteins of the retroviral capsid) (Klein, O'Neill, 2018). In the course of evolution, the specific ERV Ty3/gypsy has become the source of Arc protein. This protein is similar in biological properties to the gag retroviral gene expression product (Pastuzyn et al., 2018).

Since domestication and use for the needs of the host, the Arc gene has become highly conserved for vertebrates, playing a role in the functioning of their brain. Expression of Arc is highly dynamic in the brain in accordance with the encoding of information in neural networks. Arc gene transcript is transported to dendrites and accumulates in areas of local synaptic activity, where translation into protein occurs (Shepherd, 2018). In neurons, the Arc protein forms spatial structures resembling viral capsids that encapsulate cell mRNA. The resulting virus-like elements in the composition of extracellular vesicles are transmitted to neighboring neurons, where they are able to translate. This phenomenon is used to consolidate long-term memory (Pastuzyn et al., 2018), in the formation of which the hippocampus is involved, where the maximum activity of TEs is detected (Coufal et al., 2009; Bailie et al., 2011; Thomas, Muotri, 2012; Bachiller et al., 2017).

Based on the data listed above, it can be concluded that the observed phenomenon of intercellular neuronal interconnection using Arc has developed in evolution as a reflection of the adaptive value of the TE transcript transfer phenomenon between postmitotic cells. It is possible that when neurons exchange virus-like mRNA particles between neurons, the ability of TEs to be integrated in a site-specific manner (Sultana et al., 2017) with a change in the expression of neuron-specific genes is used to form long-term memory. As a result, the functioning of neurons and the storage of information in the brain change (Bachiller et al., 2017).

Go to:
Other functions of transposable elements

Transposable elements transpositions affect gene expression in various ways. Insertions within a gene can cause frameshift mutations, premature stop codons, or exon skipping. In the transcribed portion of the gene, TEs can reduce mRNA levels by slowing transcription due to the high A/T content in ORF2 of TEs such as L1 RE (Thomas, Muotri, 2012). However, despite the potentially mutagenic effect TEs play a role in the evolution of the genomes of all eukaryotes through the use of TE sequences to form host adaptive abilities (Mustafin, Khusnutdinova, 2019). TEs are involved in controlling the expression of protein-coding genes, many of which (Joly-Lopez, Bureau, 2018), including transcription factors (Ito et al., 2017), originated from TEs. In addition to the direct domestication of TEs, new protein-coding genes were formed due to exonization and duplication of genes using TEs (Thomas, Muotri, 2012; Joly-Lopez, Bureau, 2018; Mustafin, Khusnutdinova, 2018).

Mechanisms derived from TEs are used by the mammalian immune system to generate antibodies using the V(D)J recombination system. TEs are the source of most steroid receptors, participating in the global regulation of cell function by the hormonal system (Lapp, Hunter, 2016). Regulatory sequences, silencers, and insulators evolved from TEs (Jjingo et al., 2014; Ito et al., 2017; Schrader, Schmitz, 2018). If TEs are inserted into non-coding regions of genomes, they are used as alternative promoters, enhancers, and polyadenylation signals of genes. For example, L1s are found in non-coding regions of 80 % of human genes, the expression pattern of which depends on the density of these REs (Klein, O'Neill, 2018).

About 60 % of all SVAs in the human genome are

located in the genes or flank them within 10 kb. These SVAs are characterized as mobile CpG islands capable of upstream or downstream regulation of gene expression by recruiting transcription factors. In addition, due to the high GC content, SVAs can form alternative DNA structures, such as the G- quadruplex (characteristic of promoters of 40 % of human genes), which affects transcription (Gianfrancesco et al., 2017). Many transcription factors are immediately directed to the relationship with TEs, forming and maintaining heterochromatin (Lapp, Hunter, 2016). TEs serve as sources of cis- and transregulatory elements that coordinate the expression of groups of genes. In addition to acting as promoters that control the expression of alternative host gene isoforms, TFBS within TEs can act as enhancers in certain tissues and at certain stages of development (Garcia-Perez et al., 2016).

In evolution, TEs were the sources of a significant part of the specific sequences of the genome, as well as transcripts and proteins interacting with them. This indicates a global regulatory role of TEs, necessary for both mitosis and meiosis, and for controlling the work of cells in interphase. For example, not only spliceosomal introns (Kubiak, Makalowska, 2017), but also the Prp8 spliceosome component originated from TEs (Galej et al., 2013). Splicing enhancers and silencers are 10-nucleotide-long ncRNAs that interact with SR proteins and snRNAs. They are formed by processing transcripts of Alu retroelements (Pastor et al., 2009). TEs turned out to be sources of satellites due to the capability of site-specific insertions (McGurk, Barbash, 2018) and illegitimate recombination, followed by amplification by gene conversion (Han et al., 2016). In evolution, TEs have become sources of telomerase and telomeres (Kopera et al., 2011), as well as centromeres (Cheng, Murata, 2003; Sharma et al., 2013; Han et al., 2016) and the protein CENP/CENH3 interacting with them (Lo-pez- Flores et al., 2004; Volff, 2006). Small ncRNAs formed upon transcription of centromeric REs are involved in the regulation of these interactions (Carone et al., 2013).

Go to:

Conclusion

Less than 1.2 % of the human genome is responsible for the coding of proteins. The remaining non-coding part of the genome was largely formed due to TEs. The data on the participation of TEs in the regulation of gene switching during cell differentiation in embryogenesis, starting with the first zygote division, suggest that somatic mosaicism observed in neurons reflects the active role of TEs in neurogenesis. A number of papers have been published proving the participation of TEs in the control of differentiation of neurons. Transposable elements are sources of ncRNA, which are also important in gene switching in brain cells. The revealed role of LTRcontaining REs in the exchange of transcripts between neurons may reflect the general principle of the participation of TEs in the regulation of gene expression for the development and maintenance of brain function. The use of Arc protein for the formation of virus-like particles in the transfer of information between cells indicates the evolutionary mechanisms of TE conversion into viruses for the formation of adaptive functions. This mechanism is associated with the use of TEs to ensure the dynamism of the genomes of postmitotic cells with the possibility of their adaptive changes in response to environmental influences. The realization of this phenomenon is possible due to reverse transcription of mRNA transported between cells with site-specific insertions, the formation of somatic mosaicism of mature neurons, and a change in gene expression for memory consolidation.

Flow of cerebrospinal fluid is driven by arterial pulsations and is reduced in hypertension

Humberto Mestre [1 2], Jeffrey Tithof [3], Ting Du [1 4], Wei Song [1], Weiguo Peng [1 5], Amanda M Sweeney [1], Genaro Olveda [1], John H Thomas [3], Maiken Nedergaard [1 5], Douglas H Kelley [6]

Affiliations expand

· PMID: 30451853 PMCID: PMC6242982 DOI: 10.1038/s41467-018-07318-3

Abstract

Flow of cerebrospinal fluid (CSF) through perivascular spaces (PVSs) in the brain is important for clearance of metabolic waste. Arterial pulsations are thought to drive flow, but this has never been quantitatively shown. We used particle tracking to quantify CSF flow velocities in PVSs of live mice. CSF flow is pulsatile and driven primarily by the cardiac cycle. The speed of the arterial wall matches that of the CSF, suggesting arterial wall motion is the principal driving mechanism, via a process known as perivascular pumping. Increasing blood pressure leaves the artery diameter unchanged but changes the pulsations of the arterial wall, increasing backflow and thereby reducing net flow in the PVS. Perfusion-fixation alters the normal flow direction and causes a 10-fold reduction in PVS size. We conclude that particle tracking velocimetry enables the study of CSF flow in unprecedented detail and that studying the PVS in vivo avoids fixation artifacts.

Enteric Dopaminergic Neurons: Definition, Developmental Lineage, and Effects of Extrinsic Denervation

Z. S. Li,[1] T. D. Pham,[1] H. Tamir,[1,2] J. J. Chen,[1] and M. D. Gershon[1]

Author information Article notes Copyright and License information PMC Disclaimer

Go to:

Abstract

The existence of enteric dopaminergic neurons has been suspected; however, the innervation of the gut by sympathetic nerves, in which dopamine (DA) is the norepinephrine precursor, complicates analyses of enteric DA. We now report that transcripts encoding tyrosine hydroxylase (TH) and the DA transporter (DAT) are present in the murine bowel (small intestine > stomach or colon; proximal colon > distal colon). Because sympathetic neurons are extrinsic, transcripts encoding TH and DAT in the bowel are probably derived from intrinsic neurons. TH protein was demonstrated immunocytochemically in neuronal perikarya (submucosal >> myenteric plexus; small intestine > stomach or colon). TH, DA, and DAT immunoreactivities were coincident in subsets of neurons (submucosal > myenteric) in guinea pig and mouse intestines *in situ* and in cultured guinea pig enteric ganglia. Surgical ablation of sympathetic nerves by extrinsic denervation of loops of the bowel did not affect DAT immunoreactivity but actually increased numbers of TH-immunoreactive neurons, expression of mRNA encoding TH and DAT, and enteric DOPAC (the specific dopamine metabolite). The fetal gut contains transiently catecholaminergic (TC) cells. TC cells are the proliferating crest-derived precursors of mature neurons that are not catecholaminergic and, thus, disappear after embryonic day (E) 14 (mouse) or E15 (rat). TC cells appear early in ontogeny, and their development/survival is dependent on *mash-1* gene expression. In contrast, the intrinsic

TH-expressing neurons of the murine bowel appear late (perinatally) and are *mash-1* independent. We conclude that the enteric nervous system contains intrinsic dopaminergic neurons that arise from a *mash-1*-independent lineage of noncatecholaminergic precursors.

Keywords: dopamine, dopamine transporter, tyrosine hydroxylase, enteric nervous system, sympathetic nerves, development

Go to:

Introduction

The enteric nervous system (ENS) is larger and more complex than other regions of the PNS, reflecting the ability of the ENS to regulate enteric behavior in the absence of CNS input (Gershon et al., 1994; Gershon, 1999; Furness, 2000). Uniquely, the enteric plexuses contain intrinsic primary afferent neurons and interneurons that enable the ENS independently to mediate integrative responses to local stimuli. Many of the small molecule neurotransmitters that are found in the CNS have also been identified in the ENS. These include ACh (Steele et al., 1991; Li and Furness, 1998; Neunlist et al., 1999; Cooke, 2000; Furness, 2000; Galligan et al., 2000), norepinephrine (NE) (Leibl et al., 1999), 5-HT (Gershon, 2000), GABA (Krantis, 2000), and glutamate (Liu et al., 1997; Kirchgessner, 2001). All are the neurotransmitters of intrinsic enteric neurons, except NE, which is restricted to the enteric projections of extrinsic (sympathetic) neurons (Costa and Furness, 1984; Keast et al., 1984; Leibl et al., 1999). Although the bowel contains dopamine (DA) (Eaker et al., 1988), it has been difficult to determine whether enteric DA is present in intrinsic neurons or, because DA is the precursor of NE, in the sympathetic innervation.

Indirect evidence supports the existence of enteric dopaminergic neurons: (1) DA immunoreactivity has been reported in gastric nerve fibers, and DA is released from the corpus of the guinea pig stomach by nerve stimulation (Shichijo et al., 1997); (2) enteric DA transporter (DAT)-immunoreactive nerves have been observed (Mitsuma et al., 1998); (3) the specific DA metabolite 3,4-dihydroxyphenylacetic acid (DOPAC) has been found in mouse intestine (Eaker et al., 1988); (4) the ratio of DA to NE is higher in the bowel than in other peripheral organs (Eaker et al., 1988); (5) enteric DA is depleted by 6-hydroxydopamine (Eaker et al., 1988); and (6) pharmacological studies of transgenic mice lacking DAT have suggested that the mouse colon may normally contain inhibitory dopaminergic neurons (Walker et al., 2000). Human enteric DA and DA-immunoreactive myenteric neurons have also been reported; moreover, DA is depleted from ganglion-containing layers of the gut in Parkinson's disease, which affects dopaminergic neurons (Singaram et al., 1995).

Transiently catecholaminergic (TC) cells are abundant in the murine bowel between embryonic day (E) 11 and E14 (Baetge and Gershon, 1989). TC cells, which express tyrosine hydroxylase (TH) and dopamine β-hydroxylase (DBH), also contain and take up NE (Cochard et al., 1978; Teitelman et al., 1978, 1981; Jonakait et al., 1979; Gershon et al., 1984b). TC cells are proliferating neuronal precursors (Teitelman et al., 1981; Baetge and Gershon, 1989; Baetge et al., 1990a,b) that express and share a dependence on the transcription factor *mash-1* (Blaugrund et al., 1996). When TC cells terminally differentiate and acquire their definitive neurotransmitter, such as 5-HT, they lose TH, NE, and high-affinity uptake of NE. If enteric dopaminergic neurons exist, therefore, they would have to develop from a separate, late-arising, *mash-1*-independent neuronal lineage.

The current study was undertaken to test the hypothesis that the mouse intestine contains intrinsic dopaminergic neurons. We used immunoblots, immunocytochemistry, and reverse transcription (RT)-PCR to determine whether intrinsic enteric neurons express dopaminergic markers, including TH, DA, and DAT. Lineage was investigated by comparing perinatal wild-type and transgenic mice that lack *mash-1*. Our observations strongly support the idea that the mouse intestine contains intrinsic dopaminergic neurons that arise late in ontogeny from a *mash-1*-independent lineage of precursor cells.

Go to:

Materials and Methods

Animals and tissue preparation. Adult CD-1 mice (25-30 gm) and guinea pigs (200-350 gm) (Charles River, Wilmington, MA) of either sex were used for these studies. Transgenic mice lacking *mash-1* were obtained from Dr. David Anderson (California Institute of Technology, Pasadena, CA) and have been described previously (Guillemot et al., 1993; Lo et al., 1994; Blaugrund et al., 1996). Adult mice and guinea pigs were killed for experimental purposes by CO_2 inhalation. This procedure was approved by the Animal Care and Use Committee of Columbia University. Perinatal animals were anesthetized on ice and killed by decapitation. The brain, stomach, duodenum, ileum, and proximal and distal colon were removed from the animals and processed for molecular and histological studies. Mice that lacked the *mash-1* transcription factor were obtained from timed pregnant C57BL6/J mice carrying a null allele in the *mash-1* locus. *mash-1-/-* mice were identified by PCR analysis of a small piece of liver that was removed from each fetus, as described previously (Blaugrund et al., 1996). Fetuses were removed from pregnant dams at E17. The day at which a vaginal plug was found was designated as day 0 gestation.

RNA extraction and preparation of cDNA. The brain, stomach, duodenum, ileum, and proximal and distal colon were collected in PBS (0.9% NaCl in 0.01 m sodium phosphate buffer, pH 7.4), which had been treated with 0.1% diethyl pyrocarbonate (depc-

PBS). After the wall of each piece of gut was opened, the tissue was cleaned with depc-PBS and transferred to Trizol (Invitrogen, Carlsbad, CA) for extraction of total RNA, which was isolated according to the manufacturer's instructions and stored at -80°C for additional use. Samples of cDNA were generated by reverse transcription with 3 µg of total RNA, 0.5 µg of random hexamer primers, 0.5 mm dNTPs, 40 U of RNAsin, and 400 U of Maloney murine leukemia virus reverse transcriptase (Life Technologies), in a 30 µl reaction volume.

PCR. Pairs of oligonucleotide primers for amplification of cDNA encoding β-actin, DAT, and TH were designed from published cDNA sequences of mouse β-actin, DAT, and TH (**Table 1**). PCR reactions for DAT were performed for 35 cycles (94°C for 30 sec, 57°C for 60 sec, and 72°C for 30 sec). Because transcripts encoding β-actin and TH were abundant, only 30 cycles of amplification were used for β-actin (94°C for 30 sec, 57°C for 45 sec, and 72°C for 30 sec) and TH (94°C for 30 sec, 58°C for 60 sec, and 72°C for 30 sec). The identity of PCR products was confirmed by sequence analysis. For this purpose, PCR products were subcloned into pGEM-T Easy vectors (Promega, Madison, WI) by using the TA-cloning kit (Invitrogen, San Diego, CA). Inserts in two individual clones were sequenced by the dideoxynucleotide chain termination method (in the DNA Facility of Columbia University). The sequences of the PCR products obtained from brain and gut with the indicated primers were found to be identical to those of the corresponding GenBank sequences in cDNAs encoding mouse β-actin, DAT, and TH.

Table 1.

Sequences of primers

Primers	GenBank accession number	Primer sequence	Primer location in the sequence

		Forward, 5′-TGT TTG AGA CCT TCA ACA CC-3′	448-467
β-Actin	X03672	Reverse, 5′-CAG TAA TCT CCT TCT GCA TCC-3′	1035-1015
		Forward, 5′-CAA TTC CAC CCT CAT CAA CC-3′	134-153
DAT	AF109391	Reverse, 5′-ACG CTC AAA ATA CTC AGC AG-3′	659-640
		Forward, 5′-TAC CGA GAG GAC AGC ATT CC-3′	798-817
TH	M69200	Reverse, 5′-TTT ACA CAG CCC AAA CTC CAC-3′	1148-1128

Open in a separate window

Real-time PCR. Real-time PCR was used to quantify mRNA encoding DAT and TH in the mouse stomach, duodenum, ileum, and proximal and distal colon. The expression of DAT and TH was normalized to that of β-*actin*, a housekeeping gene that is not thought to be subject to regulation. Transcripts encoding β-actin in samples of mouse gut were first quantified by real-time PCR with the SYBR Green I kit (Roche Molecular Biochemicals, Indianapolis, IN) using a LightCycler instrument (Roche). Measurements were obtained by referring to standard curves that were prepared by serially diluting plasmid DNA encoding DAT, TH, and β-actin. The dilutions of β-actin and TH plasmid DNA ranged from 1 pg to 10 ng in five series, each of which covered a 10-fold range. Plasmid DNA encoding DAT was diluted serially from 0.01-100 pg, again in five series, each of which covered a 10-fold range.

Amplifications were performed in a final volume of 20 µl of a commercial reaction mixture (Roche) that contained *Taq*DNA polymerase, reaction buffer, dNTPs in which dTTP is replaced by dUTP, SYBR Green I dye, and $MgCl_2$. The primers for the amplification of cDNA encoding β-actin, DAT, and TH were used at a final concentration of 0.3 μm. The final concentration of $MgCl_2$ was 2.5 mm for the amplification of β-actin, 4 mm for that of DAT, and 3 mm for that of TH. To this mixture were added 2 μl of either the serial diluted plasmid DNA (standards) or the cDNA prepared from tissue. The standards and the cDNA from tissues were subjected simultaneously to real-time PCR analysis in parallel capillary tubes. Within the instrument, the reaction mixture was first incubated for at 95°C for 30 sec to denature the template DNA. Amplification was then performed for 40 cycles, each involving denaturation at 95°C for 0 sec, annealing for 5 sec at 57°C (DAT and β-actin) or 58°C (TH), and elongation at 72°C for 21 sec (DAT), 14 sec (TH), or 24 sec (β-actin). The appearance of double-stranded DNA was quantified by measuring the fluorescence of SYBR Green after each step of elongation. A melting point analysis was finally performed to improve the sensitivity and specificity of amplification reactions detected with the SYBR Green I dye; samples were incubated at 95°C for 0 sec, at 67°C for 15 sec, and then from 67 to 95°C with a transition rate of 0.2°C/sec. Data were analyzed with computer assistance using the LightCycler software.

Immunoprecipitation. Samples containing 200 μg of protein from mouse brain, stomach, duodenum, ileum, and proximal and distal colon were removed, and 10 μl of goat anti-DAT antibody (Research Diagnostics Inc., Flanders, NJ) was added in a total volume of 50 μl. After incubation at 4°C overnight, 20 μl of washed UltraLink Immobilized Protein A/G (Pierce, Rockford, IL) was added, followed by incubation at 4°C with gentle agitation overnight. The reaction mixture was washed and centrifuged at 2,000 × g for 2 min, and the supernatant was removed for DAT Western blotting.

Gel electrophoresis and immunoblotting. Tissue was harvested from mouse brain, stomach, duodenum, ileum, and proximal and distal colon, washed with PBS, and homogenized in 300 μl of 50 mm Tris buffer, pH 7.4, containing EDTA (1.0 mm), EGTA (2.0 mm), PMSF (1.0 mm), aprotinin (100 μg/ml), and leupeptin (100 μg/ml). The homogenate was centrifuged at 10,000 × g for 30 min at 4°C to separate a membrane fraction (pellet) from the cytosol. The pellet was solubilized in the same buffer containing Triton X-100 (1.0%). Proteins (50 μg) were separated by 8.5% SDS-PAGE. After separation, the proteins were electroblotted onto polyvinylidene difluride membranes and immersed in blocking buffer containing 5% nonfat dry milk in TBS for 30 min at room temperature. The blot was washed with TBS containing 0.05% Tween 20 (TBST) and finally incubated overnight at 4°C with polyclonal primary antibodies to TH, DAT, or actin (**Table 2**) (diluted 1:1000 in 3% nonfat dry milk). After washing in TBST, the blot was incubated with goat HRP-labeled secondary antibodies to rabbit IgG (Vector Laboratories, Burlingame, CA) for 1 hr at room temperature. The blot was washed with TBST and developed with a chemiluminescent substrate (Pierce, Rockford, IL).

Table 2.

Primary antibodies

		Dilution			
Antigen	Antibody	Immunocytochemistry	Western blot	Source	References
Actin	Rabbit polyclonal	N/A	1:1000	Sigma	Shanavas et al. (1996)
DA	Mouse monoclonal	1:1600	N/A	Chemicon (Temecula, CA)	Singaram et al. (1995)
DAT	Rabbit polyclonal	1:400	1:1000	Chemicon	Mitsuma et al. (1998), Lee et al. (1999)
Hu	Human	1:1500	N/A	Molecular	Marusich et

				Probes	al. (1994)	
TH	Rabbit	N/A	1:1000	Protos Biotech (New York, NY)	Pickel et al. (1980)	
TH	Sheep polyclonal	1:800	N/A	Chemicon	Li et al. (1998), Young et al. (1999)	

Open in a separate window

N/A, Not applicable.

Extrinsic denervation. The extrinsic innervation was ablated in segments of small intestine in 10 mice. The animals were anesthetized with a subcutaneous injection of a mixture of ketamine (90 mg/kg) and xylazine (5 mg/kg). The depth of anesthesia was monitored by checking the withdrawal reflex evoked by gentle squeezing of a toe with a pair of forceps. The surgical procedure used for denervation was similar to that used previously in the guinea pig small intestine (**Li et al., 1998; Pan and Gershon, 2000**). Two loops of intestine were denervated in each animal. For each denervation, a loop of ileum supplied by a single mesenteric artery and its branches was selected. On the mesenteric artery, the vessel was manipulated at a site that was 2-3 cm distant from the intestinal wall. All of the nerve fiber bundles at this site that could be seen to follow the mesenteric artery and vein that supplied the loop of the bowel were stripped away using fine forceps under microscopic control. To ablate any nerve fibers that were not severed by this procedure, the pair of vessels on the operation site were painted with a small amount of 80% phenol in distilled water, which was applied by a small swab under microscopic control. The excess phenol was then washed away thoroughly with 0.9% NaCl. The denervated region of the gut was marked by a loose ligature placed around its vascular supply, the bowel was returned to the

173

abdominal cavity, and the abdomen was closed. After surgery, pain was minimized by the subcutaneous administration of buprenorphine (1 mg/kg). The animals were then allowed to recover from anesthesia and given *ad libitum* access to food and water. The mice were killed by CO_2 inhalation 1 week after surgery. The two denervated loops of ileum and a single loop of normal small intestine (as control) were removed from each animal and analyzed by RT-PCR and immunocytochemistry. The sympathetic innervation of the gut was used as marker of the extrinsic innervation and was assessed to evaluate the extent of denervation. TH was demonstrated immunohistochemically to visualize the characteristic network of sympathetic terminals in the enteric plexuses. The denervated and control loops of gut were each divided into two equal pieces. One piece of tissue was used for RNA isolation and the other part for immunocytochemistry.

Immunocytochemistry. Segments of ileum and colon of mice and guinea pigs were collected in PBS, to which the muscle relaxant nicardipine was added to prevent spasm (10_{-6} m; Sigma, St. Louis, MO). Preparations were cut open along the mesenteric border, and the contents were flushed out with PBS. If whole mounts were to be prepared, the tissue was pinned flat on balsa wood with the mucosal surface facing down and stretched tautly. Specimens were fixed for 2 hr at room temperature with 4% formaldehye (from paraformaldehyde; pH 7.4) and washed with PBS three times for 10 min. Laminar preparations of the longitudinal muscle with attached myenteric plexus (LM-MP) and of the submucosa were obtained by dissection. Tissue to be sectioned was not stretched and was cryoprotected by infiltration with 30% sucrose in PBS containing 0.1% sodium azide overnight at 4°C. The preparations were embedded in optimal cutting temperature compound (Tissue Tek, Elkhart, IN) and cut at 10 μm with a cryostat microtome. Slides were air dried for 1 hr at room temperature. For immunostaining, specimens were permeabilized by incubation with 1% Triton X100 in PBS containing 10% normal rabbit, goat, or lamb serum (depending on the host species used to generate secondary antibodies, to block nonspecific staining) for 30 min at room temperature. Tissues were then incubated overnight with primary antibodies (Table 2) at room temperature. After being washed in PBS three times for 10 min, the tissue was incubated with appropriate affinity-purified species-specific secondary antibodies for 1-2 hr at room temperature. To demonstrate the immunoreactivity of DA, the monoamine oxidase (MAO) inhibitor pargyline was injected intraperitoneally (100 μg/kg) in mice or guinea pigs 30 min before the animals were killed (Costa and Furness, 1971) or added to the medium (100 ng/ml) of cultured myenteric neurons 1 hr before fixation. A commercial kit (Iso-IHC, Mouse on Mouse kit; InnoGenex, San Ramon, CA), which permits the use of murine antibodies to immunostain mouse tissue, was used to demonstrate DA immunoreactivity in mouse gut. The working concentrations of the secondary antibodies used for immunofluorescence were: biotin-labeled goat anti-human (Molecular Probes, Eugene, OR), goat anti-rabbit Alexa 594 (1:400; Molecular Probes), swine anti-sheep FITC (1:50; ICN Immuno Biologicals, Lisle, IL), biotin-labeled goat anti-mouse IgG (1:400; Kirkegaard & Perry Laboratories, Gaithersburg, MD), Alexa 350-labeled avidin (Molecular Probes), and FITC-labeled streptavidin (1:200; Vector Laboratories).

HPLC analysis of DA and DOPAC. Extrinsically denervated and control loops of ileum (0.5 gm, wet weight) were removed from adult CD-1 mice and homogenized in 0.5 ml 0.4 M perchloric acid ($HClO_4$). The homogenate was then centrifuged at 11,000 × g for 10 min at 4°C. The resulting supernatant was transferred to fresh microcentrifuge tubes and stored at -80°C. The supernatants were used for the assay of DA and DOPAC by HPLC (Waters Associates, Miford, MA) with electrochemical detection (Tamir et al., 1994; Liu et al., 2000).

Myenteric ganglion isolation. The ganglia of guinea pig ileum were isolated as described previously (Chen et al., 2003). Briefly, the whole length of ileum was collected in ice-cold Krebs solution. After the gut contents were washed out with Krebs solution, the ileum was kept in ice-cold MEM (Invitrogen, Carlsbad, CA) with 25 mm HEPES (Sigma). The LM-MP was then dissected mechanically from the bowel and incubated at 37°C for 1-2 hr in MEM, to which 1 mg/ml collagenase A (Boehringer Mannheim, Indianapolis, IN) and 1 mg/ml DNase I (Boehringer Mannheim) had been added. Individual myenteric ganglia were collected under microscopic control. Selected ganglia were plated in 2-well chamber slides that had been coated previously with poly-d-lysine (10 mg/ml) and mouse laminin (10 mg/ml) and cultured in a medium consisting of DMEM-F12 (Invitrogen, Gaithersburg, MD) supplemented with 2% FBS (Invitrogen), penicillin-streptomycin (1%), gentamycin (100 mg/ml; Sigma), and fungizone (5.25 mg/ml; Invitrogen). Mitotic inhibitors [5-fluoro-20-deoxyuridine (10 mm), uridine (10 mm), and cytosine β-d-arabinofuranoside (1 mm); Sigma] were added to prevent the growth of non-neuronal cells. After 1 week *in vitro*, cultures were rinsed with PBS and fixed in 4% formaldehyde (from paraformaldehyde; pH 7.4) for 30 min and processed for immunocytochemistry.

Go to:

Results

Transcripts encoding TH are found in the mouse gut

RT-PCR was used to determine whether RNA extracted from the stomach, duodenum, ileum, and proximal and distal colon contains transcripts encoding TH. The brain was studied at the same time as a positive control. mRNA encoding TH was investigated as a marker for intrinsic catecholaminergic neurons. Noradrenergic and dopaminergic neurons both contain TH; however, the murine bowel does not contain intrinsic noradrenergic neurons. The noradrenergic components of the ENS are extrinsic axons projecting from sympathetic ganglia (Costa and Furness, 1984; Keast et al., 1984; Wood, 1999). Although noradrenergic axons contain TH protein transported from cell bodies, they would not be expected to express mRNA encoding TH. Transcripts encoding TH were found in each of the examined regions of the bowel and in the brain (Fig. 1A). mRNA encoding TH was quantified in the different regions of the gut by using real-time PCR to amplify cDNA. The abundance of mRNAs encoding β-actin and TH was measured in five regions of the bowel (stomach, duodenum, ileum, and proximal and distal colon) in each of the five mice. The relative quantity of mRNA encoding TH was normalized to that encoding β-actin in each region (Fig. 1B). The relative abundance of mRNA encoding TH did not differ statistically in samples of the stomach, duodenum, ileum, and proximal colon; however, each of these regions contained significantly more mRNA encoding TH than did the distal colon ($p < 0.02$). Because the mature gut lacks noradrenergic neurons, these data are, by elimination, consistent with the idea that a subset of intrinsic cells is dopaminergic.

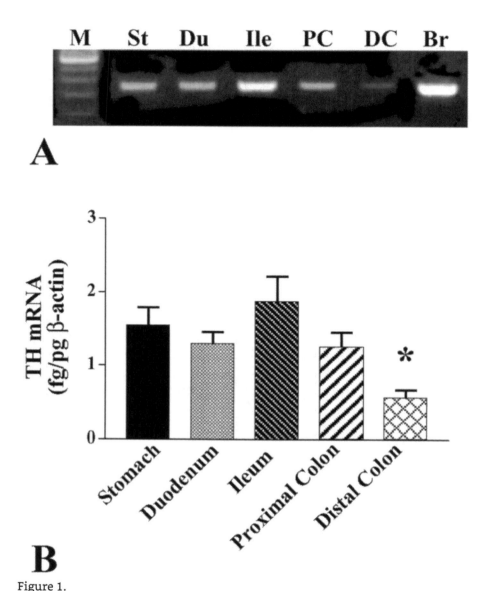

A

B

Figure 1.
Transcripts encoding TH are expressed in the mouse gut. *A*, RNA was extracted from adult mouse stomach (St), duodenum (Du), ileum (Ile), proximal colon (PC), distal colon (DC), and brain (Br), which served as a positive control, and analyzed by RT-PCR. M, 100 bp size markers. *B*, The abundance of transcripts encoding TH in each region of the bowel relative to those encoding β-actin were determined by real-time PCR. The abundance of transcripts encoding TH is significantly lower in the distal colon than in other regions of the bowel ($*p < 0.02$).

DAT is expressed in the mouse gut

The expression of transcripts encoding DAT was investigated in the murine bowel because DAT is normally restricted in its expression to dopaminergic neurons (Iversen, 2000). The gut would, therefore, be expected to express DAT if it contains intrinsic dopaminergic neurons. Prior studies, using RT-PCR, have demonstrated the presence of transcripts encoding DAT in the mouse ileum and colon (Chen et al., 2001). These transcripts were found to be absent in transgenic C57BL/6 mice that lack the gene encoding DAT; however, they were found in transgenic C57BL/6 mice that lack the serotonin transporter. We confirmed these observations in the stomach, duodenum, ileum, and proximal and distal colon of CD-1 mice. By using real-time PCR, we then evaluated quantitatively the relative expression of DAT in the stomach, duodenum, ileum, and proximal and distal colon of CD-1 mice (Fig. 2). mRNA encoding DAT was normalized to that of β-actin in each sample (Fig. 2A). Because considerable variation was encountered between animals, the values obtained in each region of the bowel were further normalized to those obtained in the duodenum of the same animal to evaluate the relative regional abundance of transcripts encoding DAT (Fig. 2B). The expression of DAT was found to be significantly higher in the duodenum than in the stomach or distal colon ($p < 0.05$). The relative abundance of mRNA encoding DAT in the intestine, thus, resembled that encoding TH in that it was least abundant in the distal colon. The presence in the gut of transcripts encoding DAT is consistent with the idea that intrinsic dopaminergic neurons exist in the bowel; however, the abundance of transcripts encoding DAT does not precisely parallel that of transcripts encoding TH.

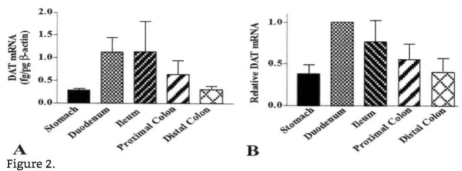

Figure 2.
Transcripts encoding DAT are expressed in the mouse gut. *A*, The abundance of transcripts encoding DAT in each region of the bowel relative to those encoding β-actin were determined by real-time PCR. *B*, The relative abundance of transcripts encoding DAT in each region of the bowel were normalized to that in the duodenum of each animal. The abundance of transcripts encoding DAT is significantly higher in the duodenum than in the stomach or distal colon (*$p <$ 0.05).

To verify that DAT protein, as well as transcripts, are expressed in the bowel, the regional distribution of DAT was analyzed by immunoblotting in the stomach, duodenum, ileum, and proximal and distal colon. TH was studied for comparison, although TH protein in extracts of gut could originate in sympathetic nerves as well as in intrinsic neurons. The brain served as a positive control, and actin was demonstrated as a loading control for the gels. Enteric DAT was concentrated by immunoprecipitation before its analysis by immunoblotting. DAT protein was detected in the stomach, duodenum, ileum, and proximal and distal colon (**Fig. 3**).

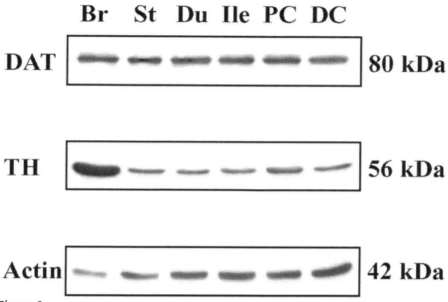

Figure 3.
DAT and TH immunoreactivities are present in the mouse gut. *A*, The distributions of DAT and TH proteins in the stomach (St), duodenum (Du), ileum (Ile), proximal colon (PC), distal colon (DC), and brain (Br) (positive control) were analyzed by immunoblotting. Enteric DAT was concentrated by immunoprecipitation before immunoblotting. Actin was analyzed as a loading control.

Coincident expression of TH and DAT immunoreactivities occurs in the ENS

DAT-immunoreactive neurons have been reported previously to be present in both the submucosal and myenteric plexuses of the mouse gut (Chen et al., 2001); however, whether or not the DAT-immunoreactive neurons in the bowel also contain TH, as would be expected of dopaminergic neurons, was not determined. We, therefore, investigated the extent to which the location of DAT immunoreactivity is coincident with that of TH in the murine ENS. The presence of DAT-immunoeactive neurons in both enteric plexuses was confirmed. DAT-immunoreactive nerve cell bodies were found to be more abundant in the submucosal than the myenteric plexus in both the ileum (Fig. 4B,E) and the colon (Fig. 4G,I). Varicose terminal axons were also DAT immunoreactive in both plexuses. DAT immunoreactivity coincided with that of TH in the cell bodies of many submucosal neurons and a smaller subset of myenteric neurons in both the ileum (Fig. 4B-F) and colon (Fig. 4G-J). Especially in the myenteric plexus, the number of varicose TH-immunoreactive axons exceeded that of DAT-immunoreactive axons, although the two markers also appeared to be colocalized in a large subset. Expression of DAT is thought to be restricted to dopaminergic neurons (Lorang et al., 1994; Ciliax et al., 1999; Holzschuh et al., 2001). DAT expression was investigated immunocytochemically in the celiac ganglion to confirm whether or not pervertebral sympathetic neurons that project to the gut are DAT immunoreactive. No DAT immunoreactivity was detected in the sympathetic neurons of the celiac ganglion (Fig. 4K), although these noradrenergic neurons were all TH immunoreactive (Fig. 4L). Because sympathetic neurons, thus, express TH but not DAT, the axons in the gut that contained TH, but not DAT, immunoreactivity were probably sympathetic. The enteric TH-immunoreactive cell bodies that also contained DAT, however, were clearly intrinsic and, thus, good candidates to be intrinsic dopaminergic neurons. Another subset of DAT-immunoreactive nerve cell bodies was observed in the myenteric plexus, however, that contained no detectable TH immunoreactivity (Fig. 4I,J). The relative numbers of DAT- and TH-immunoreactive neurons were quantified in the myenteric and submucosal plexuses of the mouse ileum. Approximately 67% of DAT-immunoreactive myenteric neurons and 64% of DAT-immunoreactive submucosal neurons were found to contain TH immunoreactivity (Table 3), and ~58% of TH-immunoreactive myenteric neurons and 65% of TH-immunoreactive submucosal neurons were found to contain DAT immunoreactivity (Table 3). The neuronal marker, Hu, was used to demonstrate immunocytochemically all enteric neurons in triply labeled preparations to quantify the proportion of enteric neurons that are DAT or TH immunoreactive. DAT-immunoreactive neurons were found to constitute ~ 10% of myenteric and 12% of submucosal neurons, whereas, TH-immunoreactive neurons constituted ~ 9% of myenteric and 13% of submucosal neurons (Table 3). DAT immunoreactivity was also examined in cryostat sections of the bowel to determine the distribution of DAT-immunoreactive fibers in layers of the gut. No fibers were detected in the muscle layers of the gut or in the mucosa (data not shown). These observations suggest that DAT-immunoreactive axons are confined to the enteric plexuses and that their targets are, thus, likely to be other enteric neurons or axons.

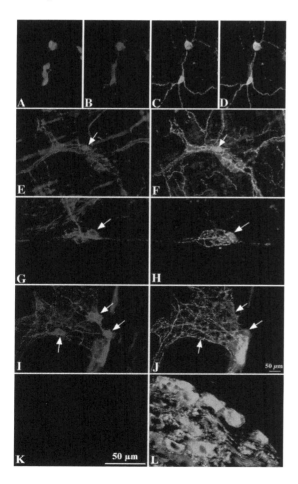

Figure 4.

DAT and TH immunoreactivities are partially coincident in the mouse ileum and colon; sympathetic neurons of the celiac ganglion are TH immunoreactive but not DAT immunoreactive. Double-label or triple immunocytochemistry illuminated to reveal Hu (*A*; blue fluorescence), DAT (*B, E, G, I, K*; red fluorescence), and TH (*C, F, H, J, L*; green fluorescence) immunoreactivities in the same fields in submucosal and myenteric plexuses of the ileum and colon. Coincident labeling is apparent in the yellow cells in the merged image of TH and DAT immunoreactivities (*D*). The immunoreactivity of Hu was studied as a neuronal marker. *A-D*, Submucosal plexus of the ileum. *E, F*, Myenteric plexus of the ileum. *G, H*, Submucosal plexus of the colon. *I, J*, Myenteric plexus of the colon. *K, L*, Celiac (prevertebral sympathetic) ganglion. Arrows indicate the locations of individual cells in paired figures. Scale bar, 50 μm.

Table 3.

Colocalization of TH and DAT immunoreactivities in the ENS

Mouse ileum	Myenteric plexus	Submucosal plexus
TH/100 DAT neurons	67 ± 9%	64 ± 11%
TH/100 neurons (total = Hu immunoreactive)	9 ± 3%	13 ± 1%
DAT/100 TH neurons	58 ± 18%	65 ± 2%
DAT/100 neurons (total = Hu immunoreactive)	10 ± 4%	12 ± 4%

Open in a separate window

Data are expressed as means ±SE. Two hundred neurons were counted in each of three mice.

Coincident expression of DA and DAT immunoreactivities occurs in the ENS

Nerve terminals containing DA immunoreactivity have been reported previously to contact choline acetyltransferase-immunoreactive neurons in the guinea pig stomach (**Shichijo et al., 1997**), and DA-immunoreactive neurons have been observed in the human (**Singaram** et al., **1995**), but not the mouse, gut. The location of DA immunoreactivity was, therefore, investigated in both the mouse and guinea pig bowel, and the extent to which DA immunoreactivity was coincident with that of DAT was also studied. The guinea pig was examined because the guinea pig ENS has been more thoroughly characterized than that of any other species. In addition, it is relatively easy to isolate and culture myenteric ganglia from guinea pigs to obtain ganglia that are free of extrinsic nerve fibers. DA-immunoreactive nerve cell bodies were found in both the submucosal and myenteric plexuses of the ileum in both mice (**Fig. 5A-D**) and guinea pigs (**Fig. 5E-H**). DA and DAT were found to be fully colocalized in neuronal perikaya in both species (over 300 neurons were analyzed in each). To be absolutely certain that the neurons that coexpressed DA and DAT were intrinsic, myenteric ganglia were isolated from the guinea pig ileum and cultured for 1 week before examination. Extrinsic elements of the ENS degenerate under these conditions. DA and DAT immunoreactivities were also found to be completely coincident in the cell bodies of the cultured myenteric neurons (**Fig. 6**). These observations suggest that DA is located in enteric neurons that express DAT and that all enteric DAT is located in intrinsic neurons, in these preparations.

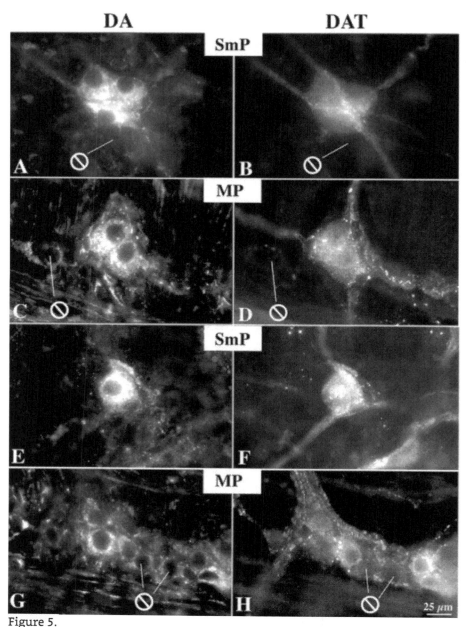

Figure 5.

DA and DAT immunoreactivities are coincident in neurons of the mouse and guinea pig ileum. Double-label immunocytochemistry illuminated to reveal DA (left; Alexa 596) and DAT immunoreactivities (right; Alexa 488) in the same fields in submucosal plexus (SmP) and myenteric plexus (MP) of the mouse (*A-D*) and guinea pig (*E-H*) ileum. DA immunoreactivity in nerve cell bodies is greater than that in fibers. ⊖, Location of neurons that lack immunoreactivity. Scale bar, 25 μm.

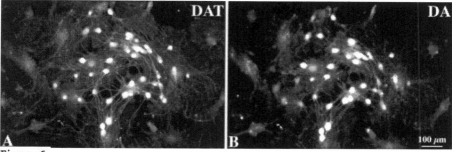

Figure 6.
DA and DAT immunoreactivities are fully coincident in nerve cell bodies in cultured myenteric ganglia isolated from guinea pig ileum. Cultures were maintained for 1 week to allow extrinsic axons to degenerate. Scale bar, 100 μm.

Extrinsic denervation increases the number of detectable TH-immunoreactive neurons in the submucosa plexus

The mouse ileum was subjected to extrinsic denervation to verify that the cells that express TH and DAT are intrinsic cells of the bowel wall and to determine whether the expression of TH by intrinsic neurons is altered by the loss of an extrinsic source of TH. Extrinsic denervation was achieved by compressing perivascular nerves in mesenteric arcades and confirmed by examining the distribution of sympathetic axons in the gut wall. After denervation, both myenteric and submucosal neuronal cell bodies continued to be both TH and DAT immunoreactive (**Fig. 7**), although the numbers of such cells were far greater in the submucosal than the myenteric plexus. In contrast, the TH-immunoreactive varicose axons, which form a dense network in the enteric plexuses of control preparations (**Fig. 7 A, E**), disappeared after denervation (**Fig. 7C,D,F**). Partial denervation was evident in the tissue at the border between fully denervated and normally innervated segments of tissue, forming an easily recognized transitional zone that permitted the precise demarcation of denervated and innervated bowel (**Fig.** 7*B*). DAT-immunoreactive cells also persisted after extrinsic denervation in both the myenteric (**Fig.** 7*G*) and submucosal plexuses (**Fig.** 7*H*). Surprisingly, TH-immunoreactive nerve cell bodies not only persisted after denervation of the gut, but their numbers increased greatly (**Fig.** 7, compare *E,F*). The number of TH-immunoreactive neurons in extrinsically denervated segments of submucosal plexus was almost threefold that of the normally innervated segments of the same bowel (**Table 4**). In contrast, the total numbers of neurons (measured either per ganglion or per unit area of tissue) were unchanged by denervation. These data suggest that the increase in number of TH-immunoreactive neurons after denervation is unlikely to be attributable to the generation of new neurons from stem cells and is probably the result of increased TH expression by existing neurons, which increases the number of cells that contain enough TH protein to be immunocytochemically detectable.

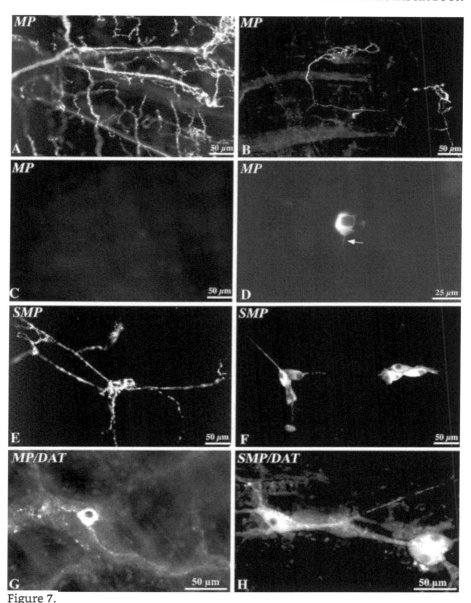

Figure 7.

Extrinsic denervation confirms that myenteric and submucosal TH-immunoreactive neurons are intrinsic. TH immunoreactivity demonstrated in laminar preparations of myenteric and submucosal plexuses. *A*, Myenteric plexus control. The sympathetic axons are characterized by large varicosities and are very abundant. *B*, Myenteric plexus at the border between denervated and innervated segments. A small number of varicose sympathetic axons remain in irregular clusters. *C*, Myenteric plexus within the denervated segment. No TH-immunoreactive sympathetic axons remain. *D*, Myenteric plexus within the denervated segment. An intrinsic TH-immunoreactive neuron can be discerned. Note the very fine axon extending from it. *E*, Submucosal plexus control. Sympathetic axons are again characterized by large varicosities. *F*, Submucosal plexus within the denervated segment. Several intrinsic TH-immunoreactive neurons can be discerned. Note their extension of fine nonvaricose axons. The varicose sympathetic axons are no longer visible. *G*, Myenteric plexus within the denervated segment showing DAT immunoreactivity. A DAT-immunoreactive neuron is apparent within a ganglion. *H*, Submucosal plexus within the denervated segment showing several DAT-immunoreactive neurons in interconnected ganglia. Scale bars: *A-C, E-H*, 50 μm; *D*, 25 μm.

Table 4.

Effect of extrinsic denervation on submucosa neurons

Parameter measured	Innervated	Denervated
TH/100 neurons (total = Hu immunoreactive)	13 ± 1	34 ± 3
Total neurons/100 ganglia	305 ± 5	289 ± 7
Neurons /2 mm2 submucosal plexus	147 ± 26	149 ± 19

Open in a separate window

Data are expressed as means ±SE (*n* = 3).

Extrinsic denervation increases the enteric expression of mRNA encoding TH and DAT

The denervation-induced increase in neurons containing immunocytochemically detectable TH could be explained by a corresponding increase in denervation-induced TH transcription. Alternatively, denervation could unmask a previously sequestered source of preexistent TH. Transcripts encoding TH were, thus, quantified by using real-time RT-PCR in extrinsically denervated and innervated segments of the bowel. Transcripts encoding DAT were also quantified to determine whether changes, if any, were restricted to transcription of TH or whether they extended also to other molecules involved in dopaminergic signaling. Extrinsic denervation of the mouse ileum was found to increase both the amount of mRNA encoding TH and that encoding DAT. RNA was extracted from the denervated and innervated segments of the bowel in eight animals, and real-time PCR was used for quantitation. The normally innervated segment of gut served as a control for the effect of extrinsic denervation in the same animal, and measured quantities of mRNA were normalized to that of β-actin in the same samples. The differences, compared by means of a paired t test, were significant both for mRNA encoding TH (control, 0.17 ±0.05; denervated, 0.45 ±0.06; $p < 0.03$) and DAT (control, 0.040 ±0.005; denervated, 0.070 ±0.008; $p < 0.02$). These data are consistent with the idea that intrinsic enteric neurons that express both TH and DAT respond to extrinsic denervation by increasing transcription of molecules associated with neurotransmitter biosynthesis and uptake. Conceivably, this upregulation is a compensatory mechanism that helps to mitigate the loss of NE.

Effects of extrinsic denervation on enteric DA and DOPAC

The increased transcription of TH and DAT in the denervated bowel suggests that the content, turnover, or both of DA should rise in the affected region. The levels of DA and its specific metabolite, DOPAC, were, therefore, measured in paired segments of innervated and denervated ileum. The pairs were obtained from the same bowel; however, they were taken from segments of gut that were vascularized by different, nonoverlapping vascular arcades, separated from each other by ~5 cm of tissue. Levels of DOPAC and DA were measured in denervated and innervated segments of the bowel in 10 animals. The normally innervated segment of gut served as a control for the effect of extrinsic denervation in the same animal. Extrinsic denervation was found to significantly increase the tissue content of DOPAC in the ileum (control, 0.45 ±0.12 pmol/mg; denervated, 0.68 ±0.17; $p < 0.05$); however, the increase in the concentration of DA in the same denervated segments of the bowel did not achieve significance (control, 0.16 ± 0.03; denervated, 0.19 ±0.13). These observations confirm that the majority of the DA in the bowel is not of sympathetic origin because the concentration of DA does not decrease when the sympathetic nerves degenerate. The increased tissue content of DOPAC in the extrinsically denervated bowel is consistent with the idea that the turnover of DA increases after denervation, possibly because dopaminergic neurons become more active; however, as usually occurs when catecholaminergic neurons are stimulated, an increase in transmitter biosynthesis compensates for the stimulation-induced transmitter release to maintain near constancy in the stores of the transmitter (Weiner, 1970; Molinoff and Axelrod, 1971; Iuvone et al., 1978).

TH neurons are present in transgenic mice that lack mash-1

TH is expressed in catecholaminergic cells in developing ENS during fetal life (Cochard et al., 1978; Teitelman et al., 1978, 1981; Jonakait et al., 1979; Gershon et al., 1984b). Expression of TH and other catecholamine-related molecules disappears from the rat gut at E15 (Baetge et al., 1990a) and from the mouse gut at E14 (Baetge et al., 1990b). These molecules disappear because the TC cells that express them are proliferating neuronal precursors that give rise to terminally differentiated neurons, such as those that express 5-HT (Teitelman et al., 1981; Gershon et al., 1984a; Baetge et al., 1990a) and nitric oxide synthase (NOS) (Branchek and Gershon, 1989; Young et al., 1999), which are not catecholaminergic. TC cells express the transcription factor Mash-1 and fail to develop when *mash-1* is deleted (Blaugrund et al., 1996); however, the possibility that a second population of catecholaminergic cells develops in the gut later in ontogeny, from Mash-1-independent precursors, after the initial Mash-1-dependent population no longer expresses TH, has not previously been investigated. Because catecholaminergic cells are present in fetal life, we tested the hypothesis that the TH-expressing dopaminergic neurons of the mature bowel arise from TC cell precursors. The expression of TH was investigated by immunocytochemistry in the bowel of wild-type (*mash-1+/+*) and transgenic mice that lack Mash-1 (*mash-1-/-*). The gut was studied in perinatal animals because *mash-1-/-* mice do not survive postnatally. Although TH disappears from the fetal mouse intestine by E14-E15 (**Baetge and Gershon, 1989**), a second late-arising population of TH-immunoreactive neurons was found to be present in the gut of wild-type mice (data not shown). In contrast to TC cells, which are found in the outer gut mesenchyme, and external to the circular muscle when that layer develops, the late-arising TH-immunoreactive cells were primarily submucosal in location. TH-immunoreactive neurons were found in the intestine both in perinatal *mash-1+/+* (0.18 cells/mm2) and perinatal *mash-1-/-* mice (2.1 cells/mm2) (**Fig. 8**). These observations indicate that the hypothesis that TC cells give rise to the dopaminergic neurons of adults can be rejected. They also suggest that a second wave of catecholaminergic neurons, which is independent of *mash-1* expression, arises perinatally. The apparent increase in packing density of TH-immunoreactive cells in *mash-1-/-* mice is likely to reflect the absence in these animals of all of those neurons that are derived from TC cell precursors. The bowel of mice that lack *mash-1* contains only Mash-1-independent neurons, such as those that contain calcitonin gene-related peptide, but not neurons that are Mash-1 dependent, such as those that contain 5-HT (**Blaugrund et al., 1996**).

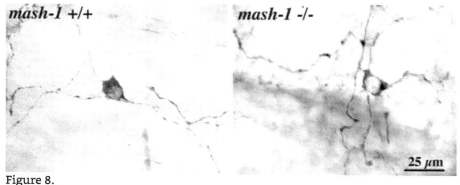

Figure 8.
TH-immunoreactive neurons are present in the bowel of transgenic mice that lack *mash-1*.

Go to:

Discussion

Observations made during the course of the present study strongly support the hypothesis that the gut contains intrinsic dopaminergic neurons. Transcripts encoding the critical biosynthetic enzyme TH are found in the bowel, and a subset of intrinsic enteric neurons is TH immunoreactive. The gut also contains mRNA encoding DAT and DAT-immunoreactive neurons. The immunoreactivities of TH and DAT colocalize in enteric neurons, which persist when enteric ganglia from the guinea pig intestine are cultured, confirming that these neurons are intrinsic. DA immunoreactivity is present in enteric neurons, colocalizes in subsets with the immunoreactivities of TH and DAT, and in cultured neurons, the immunoreactivity of DA is absolutely coincident with that of DAT. Neurons that contain TH and DAT can potentially obtain DA by synthesizing it from tyrosine or by taking it up from the ambient medium. TH is the rate-limiting enzyme in DA biosynthesis, but aromatic l-amino acid decarboxylase is also required to convert l-dihydroxyphenylalanine (l-DOPA) to DA.

Intrinsic neurons of the bowel that contain aromatic l-amino acid decarboxylase have long been known to be present in the ENS. These cells, which were found to be more numerous in the submucosal than the myenteric plexus, were originally called "amine handling neurons" because they synthesize DA from l-DOPA and 5-HT from 5-hydroxytryptophan (Costa et al., 1976; Furness and Costa, 1978; Furness et al., 1980). The distribution of amine handling neurons (Furness and Costa, 1978) is similar to that of the TH-immunoreactive neurons of the mouse intestine. Because they are DA immunoreactive in the absence of pretreatment with exogenous l-DOPA or DA, the intrinsic neurons found in the current study to contain the immunoreactivities of TH and DAT probably also contain aromatic l-amino acid decarboxylase. These intrinsic TH-, DA-, and DAT-immunoreactive neurons are, thus, likely to have been included in, or identical to, the population of amine handling neurons described previously. Intrinsic enteric neurons, thus, contain DA, contain the enzymes needed to synthesize it from tyrosine, and can inactivate DA (by DAT-mediated reuptake) after its release from stimulated neurons. Given that DA is also released from stimulated enteric neurons (Shichijo et al., 1997) and exerts effects on enteric neurons (Hirst and Silinsky, 1975) and neurites that are identical pharmacologically to those of an endogenous transmitter (Kusunoki et al., 1985), DA fulfills the criteria necessary to identify it as an enteric neurotransmitter (Iversen, 1979).

In addition to the neurons in which the immunoreactivities of TH and DAT colocalize, the gut also contains a small number of neurons that contain the immunoreactivity of DAT, but not that of TH; moreover, the relative abundance of transcripts encoding TH and DAT is not identical in all regions of the bowel. It is possible that a subset of noncatecholaminergic enteric neurons contains DAT; however, this possibility is not supported by the observation that every neuron found *in vitro* to contain DAT also contains DA. Conceivably, the DA in some DAT-expressing neurons reflects the uptake of DA produced by another cell in the cultures. No DA was added to the incubation medium, however, and DA is highly unstable in solutions that lack antioxidants. It, thus, seems more likely that the DA immunoreactivity found in DAT-immunoreactive neurons *in vitro* reflects the biosynthesis of DA by these cells. Alternatively, DAT could be found in neurons that apparently lack TH if the level of TH were to vary according to physiological circumstances in individual neurons, so as to rise above or fall below the threshold necessary for immunocytochemical detection. If this alternative is correct, then the gut might contain a fixed number of potentially dopaminergic neurons (at least some of which are DAT immunoreactive) that is greater than the number that is demonstrated with antibodies to TH. The number of neurons that are functionally dopaminergic may be submaximal until the bowel is stressed by circumstances that provoke the upregulation of TH.

Extrinsic denervation may be an example of a stimulus that upregulates TH and other molecules related to dopaminergic mechanisms. Extrinsic denervation increases both the abundance of transcripts encoding both TH and DAT in the bowel and leads to a threefold increase in the numbers of demonstrable TH-immunoreactive enteric neurons. These neurons, moreover, appear in the absence of a corresponding increase in the total numbers of neurons in either enteric plexus. The increment in TH-immunoreactive neurons, thus, appears to be the result of recruitment of existing neurons to the dopaminergic phenotype, rather than the *de novo* genesis of new neurons from stem cells, although stem cells do exist in the mature bowel (Bixby et al., 2002; Kruger et al., 2002).

The upregulation of TH and DAT induced by extrinsic denervation is not accompanied by an increase in the DA concentration of the intestine. Instead, extrinsic denervation leads to an increase in the concentration of DOPAC, the specific metabolite of DA. The persistence of DA and DOPAC in the extrinsically denervated bowel clearly establishes that sympathetic nerves are responsible neither for the bulk of the DA stored in the gut nor for its metabolism by MAO. In contrast, the increase in the metabolism of DA to DOPAC that occurs when sympathetic or other extrinsic nerves are absent is consistent with the idea that extrinsic denervation provokes an increase in the activity of intrinsic dopaminergic neurons. Release and DAT-mediated reuptake of DA by activated neurons would be expected to mobilize sequestered DA from storage vesicles and, thus, enhance its metabolism by promoting exposure of DA to mitochondrial MAO. Increased activity of dopaminergic neurons in other locations has also been found to be associated with increased biosynthesis of DA (Iuvone et al., 1978), which would account, in the ENS, for the extrinsic denervation-induced upregulation in transcription of TH. Transmitter content normally remains relatively constant in catecholaminergic neurons, despite marked fluctuations in neuronal activity (Weiner, 1970; Molinoff and Axelrod, 1971).

It is not clear how extrinsic denervation increases dopaminergic activity in the ENS. Extrinsic sympathetic nerves are known to decrease the release of ACh from excitatory cholinergic nerve terminals *via* α-2 adrenoceptors (Scheibner et al., 2002) and to evoke IPSPs in submucosal neurons (Wood, 1999). The effects of DA on enteric neurons have not been investigated thoroughly, but, like NE, DA is known to inhibit the release of ACh from stimulated enteric nerves (Kusunoki et al., 1985), and DA also mimics the effects on submucosal neurons of NE and sympathetic nerve stimulation (Hirst and Silinsky, 1975). The net effects on the ENS of DA released from intrinsic dopaminergic neurons and NE released from extrinsic sympathetic nerve terminals may, thus, be similar. If so, the upregulation of dopaminergic mechanisms might help to compensate for the loss of the extrinsic sympathetic innervation. In fact, a previous study noted that extrinsic denervation increases the intestinal content of aromatic amino acid decarboxylase and speculated that sympathetic nerves exert "some restraining influence" on the amine handling neurons that contain this enzyme (Mann et al., 1989). The mechanism that functionally couples the extrinsic sympathetic and intrinsic dopaminergic innervations of the bowel remains to be determined. Also remaining to be ascertained is the identity of inputs to enteric dopaminergic neurons, the neuroactive substances, if any, that are co-stored with DA, and the enteric circuits in which dopaminergic neurons function.

The development of enteric dopaminergic neurons is somewhat surprising in that they appear to arise independently of the catecholaminergic precursors that are found in the early fetal bowel. These TC precursors, which are *mash-1* dependent, proliferate and characteristically give rise to terminally differentiated neurons that are born early in the ontogeny of the bowel, including those that contain 5-HT or NOS (Branchek and Gershon, 1989; Pham et al., 1991; Blaugrund et al., 1996; Young et al., 1999). Although TC cells express TH, they appear to contain NE rather than DA, and because they specifically take up 3H-NE (Gershon et al., 1984b), they evidently express the NE transporter rather than DAT. In contrast, dopaminergic neurons arise perinatally, which is relatively late in the development of the ENS (Pham et al., 1991), and like other late-developing neurons (Branchek and Gershon, 1989; Pham et al., 1991; Blaugrund et al., 1996; Young et al., 1999), dopaminergic neurons appear to be *mash-1* independent. The function of the expression of catecholaminergic properties in enteric neuronal precursor cells has never been ascertained, although it might be related to a still-to-be-determined developmental role played by NE. Mice that lack TH (Thomas et al., 1995; Zhou et al., 1995) or DBH (Thomas et al., 1995) exhibit similar patterns of fetal lethality, whereas mice that lack DA, but not NE, are viable (Zhou and Palmiter, 1995). NE, but not DA, is, thus, essential for viability in fetal mice (Thomas et al., 1995). The necessary role played by NE in fetal development is compatible with the possibility that NE exerts trophic effects during development (Zhou et al., 1995). If so, then NE from TC cells could be an enteric trophic factor; however, fetal NE may be required simply to maintain heart rate during periods of stress (Portbury et al., 2003). Whatever the role of NE from TC cells may be, neither NE nor TC cells or their progeny are needed for the development of enteric dopaminergic neurons, which develop normally in the TC cell-deficient bowel of mash-1-/- mice.

Made in the USA
Middletown, DE
27 June 2024

56481561R00135